NORMAL ANATOMY
FOR
MULTIPLANAR IMAGING
Head, Neck, and Spine

NORMAL ANATOMY FOR MULTIPLANAR IMAGING
Head, Neck, and Spine

Bharat Raval, M.D.

Associate Professor
Department of Radiology
University of Texas Medical School
Houston, Texas

Joel W. Yeakley, M.D.

Assistant Professor
Department of Radiology
University of Texas Medical School
Houston, Texas

John H. Harris, Jr., M.D., D.Sc.

Professor and Chairman
Department of Radiology
University of Texas Medical School
Houston, Texas

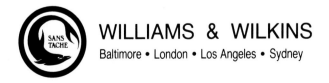

WILLIAMS & WILKINS
Baltimore • London • Los Angeles • Sydney

Editor: Timothy H. Grayson
Associate Editor: Carol Eckhart
Copy Editor: Linda Hansford
Design: JoAnne Janowiak
Illustration Planning: Wayne Hubbel
Production: Anne G. Seitz

Printed in the United States of America

Library of Congress Cataloging-in-Publication Data

Raval, Bharat.
    Normal anatomy for multiplanar imaging.

    Bibliography: p.
    1. Head—Anatomy—Atlases. 2. Neck—Anatomy—Atlases. 3. Spine—Anatomy—Atlases. 4. Diagnostic imaging—Atlases. I. Yeakley, Joel W. II. Harris, John H., 1925-. III. Title. [DNLM: 1. Head—anatomy & histology. 2. Head—radiography. 3. Neck—anatomy & histology. 4. Neck—radiography. 5. Spine—anatomy & histology. 6. Spine—radiography. WE 705 R252n]
QM535.R37 1987   611'.91   86-26700
ISBN 0-683-07153-X

Composed and printed at the   87 88 89 90 91
Waverly Press, Inc.   10 9 8 7 6 5 4 3 2 1

To our families and our teachers.

BHARAT RAVAL, M.D.
JOEL W. YEAKLEY, M.D.
JOHN H. HARRIS, JR., M.D., D.SC.

Foreword

Teaching of generic anatomy in today's medical school curricula provides a useful introduction to specialized anatomic knowledge required by individual medical, surgical, and radiologic disciplines. During their radiologic residencies, most physicians struggled to conceptualize three-dimensional anatomy from integrated two-dimensional images. No sooner was a reasonable comfort level obtained than multiple cross-sectional and multiplanar imaging modalities sent them scurrying back to the study of pre-19th century atlases or morbid anatomy.

Shortly after the introduction of computed tomography, a number of useful atlases appeared that directly compared CT cross-sectional images with anatomic drawings and photographs of cadaver cross-sections; their scope was usually limited to the brain and torso. As helpful as these efforts were, they were handicapped almost immediately by changing technology that produced better image quality and, subsequently, sagittal and coronal reformatting of the axial images.

Magnetic resonance imaging was introduced with the CT axial anatomic foundation developed, but with a new complexity arising from direct coronal and sagittal acquisitions—primary multiplanar imaging.

This book is organized in an atlas form with side-by-side CT or MRI images and anatomic line drawings of the images on which considerable anatomic detail is labeled but which is pertinent to the clinical image interpretation. The reader can study the images first, then check anatomic knowledge against the diagrams. For clinical practice, unknown or uncertain structures identified on images can be referenced to the line drawings.

The sections on the sella turcica, orbits, paranasal sinuses, nasopharynx, temporal bone, and extremities are particularly useful in defining the anatomy of the more infrequently performed examinations.

This text represents a monumental effort to bring together anatomic comparisons of the entire body that will be largely independent of changing technology. From the brain to the extremities, the authors have succeeded in producing a text for a range of audiences. Medical students, radiology residents, practitioners, specialists, and generalists alike will find not only a complete and enduring reference, but a self-study guide as well.

Thomas F. Meaney, M.D., F.A.C.R.
Chairman, Department of Radiology
Cleveland Clinic Foundation
Cleveland, Ohio

Preface

The preparation of a radiologic anatomic atlas of the entire body is an enormous undertaking which requires the timely integration of several disparate but essential factors. These include proven clinical experience to provide the basic knowledge to be shared and sufficient material to provide a source of appropriate illustrations; a strong motivation for teaching; dedication to the task and the commitment of a remarkable amount of time and energy on the part of the authors; and a talented, interested medical illustrator. Given these conditions, there is a reasonable probability that the concept will come to successful fruition. The confluence of these factors has resulted in the publication of this text "Normal Anatomy for Multiplanar Imaging."

The motivation to prepare this text arose from the perceived need for a comprehensive atlas for multiplanar anatomy of the entire body. The goal was to design a format which included a sufficient number of appropriate images so that the atlas would be useful to generally practicing as well as academic radiologists, to radiology residents, and to practitioners and residents of those medical disciplines that have a need to understand multiplanar imaging. It is our sincere hope that our combined private practice and academic radiologic experience has enabled us to mold the text so as to achieve this goal.

Since the authors have a significant role in the preparation of a textbook, it is with great personal pleasure and professional pride that I introduce the principal authors of this text, who are both my friends and associates, to you, the reader.

Bharat Raval, M.D., Associate Professor of Radiology, began his academic career in 1978 at the University of Western Ontario under the very capable leadership and tutelage of Lewis S. Carey, M.D., Professor and Chairman of the Department of Radiology at that Institution. Dr. Raval has done abdominal imaging all of his professional life, and introduced many of the sophisticated diagnostic and interventional procedures related to the alimentary tract and its adjacent organ systems at the University of Western Ontario. In 1982, Dr. Raval joined the faculty of the University of Texas Medical School at Houston and the Hermann Hospital, where he has continued to develop his already considerable abilities in teaching and diagnostic abdominal imaging. His interest and ability in ultrasound and body CT are internationally recognized. Dr. Raval's talents, interests, and dedication are evidenced in all of the nonneuroradiologic portions of this text.

Joel W. Yeakley, M.D., Assistant Professor of Radiology, entered the private practice of radiology, with an emphasis in neuroradiology, in 1976 following resident training in both neurology and radiology at the University of Florida, Gainsville. In 1982, he became a Fellow in Neuroradiology at the University of Texas Medical School at Houston and the Hermann Hospital and, enticed by the stimulation and excitement of this academic environment, has stayed on our faculty. Dr. Yeakley, under the guidance and stimulation of K. Francis Lee, M.D., D.Sc., Professor and Chief of Neuroradiology, not only has become an excellent academic neuroradiologist, but has developed a particular interest in the sella and the parasellar structures. Through his own initiative, and stimulated by the patient volume of a very sophisticated Department of Oto-Rhino-Laryngology, Dr. Yeakley has become an authority on imaging of the temporal bone. These special interests are reflected in the neuroradiologic portion of this text, which was prepared by Dr. Yeakley.

Juan A. Cabrera, M.D., Assistant Professor of Neurosurgery at the University of Texas Medical School at Houston and the Hermann Hospital, prepared the line drawing of each multiplanar image only after close and detailed collaboration with the authors. The precision of Dr. Cabrera's drawings highlights and clarifies the frequently complex anatomy so exquisitely displayed by the GE 9800 CT and Signa System MR images. Thus Dr. Cabrera's participation in this work has been more than that of simply a medical illustrator, and his contributions to the neuroradiologic portion of the atlas have been extremely valuable.

Each of the CT or MR images in the atlas was specifically selected by the authors to illustrate particular radiologic anatomy. Each image was selected after critical review of literally hundreds of similar images. The anatomic structures to be identified on each drawing were also specifically indicated by the authors.

The format of line drawing and multiplanar image on facing pages was selected to facilitate visual correlation of the labeled drawing and the image, uncluttered by labels or lines. Where possible, the multiplanar images have been reproduced in the same size as used in daily practice.

Because this text was designed to be an atlas of multiplanar anatomy and because of the quality of the images and the explanatory nature of the line drawings of each specific image, we consider the labeled drawing to be the "legend" of each figure. In like fashion, we decided that the high resolution images provided a more eloquent display of normal multiplanar anatomy than would be possible by any narrative. Consequently, the narrative portion of this text has been kept as brief as possible to allow the illustrations to speak for themselves.

It is our sincere hope and intention that this atlas become a useful reference to those using multiplanar imaging, and that the ultimate result of the time, energy, and effort of all concerned in the preparation of this text be improved patient care.

John H. Harris Jr., M.D., D.Sc.
Professor and Chairman
Department of Radiology
University of Texas Medical School
Houston, Texas

Acknowledgments

We freely acknowledge that this atlas could not have been considered, let alone completed, without the interest and dedication of our secretaries: Margaret Pirtle, Carol Hitchcock, Sandra Sundve, Kathy Norred, and Toni Jones-Tate.

The benchmark of any atlas is the quality of the illustrations. In this regard, we are indebted to General Electric Medical Systems for the exquisite quality and resolution of the images which were all obtained from GE 9800 CT scanners and a 1.5 T Signa MR System. GE Medical Systems has been, and continues to be, a positive and supportive influence in the activities of this Department. Their support of, and participation in, the completion of this atlas is yet another example of the altruism of the Medical Systems division of General Electric. In this regard, we are particularly indebted to Robert L. Stocking, Vice President and General Manager, Sales and Service Division, Steven B. Leadley, Sales Manager, and Christine Capitan, Sales Representative.

The faithful reproduction of the high quality and definition in the illustrations of this atlas is a tribute to the photographic capability of Jay Johnson, B.S., Medical Photographer of the Department of Radiology.

The Hermann Hospital CT technologists, Yvonne Stuart, Pat Simpson, Jesus Cagigal, Kinnon Bell, Mike Millis, Veronica Dolney, and Larry Abdella, under the supervision of Gilberto Garza, R.T., and the MR technologists of The University of Texas Medical School at Houston, Elizabeth Berry, Terry Etheredge, and Steven M. Blackburn, merit our appreciation in obtaining the images which are the essence of this atlas.

Madan V. Kulkarni, M.D., Director of MR at The University of Texas Medical School at Houston and the Hermann Hospital, gave freely of his time and considerable ability in the selection of the MR images.

Finally, we are proud to acknowledge the assistance, support, and encouragement of Carol Eckhart, Associate Editor, and Timothy Grayson, Editor, and the very cordial and professional good offices of Williams & Wilkins in the design and production of this atlas.

Contents

1

Skull and Brain

BRAIN

SKULL BASE

CISTERNOGRAM

Axial CT examinations of the brain are usually performed at an angle of approximately +25° to Reid's base line. Images obtained parallel to Reid's base line may provide a better view of the posterior fossa. Images obtained in planes perpendicular to or parallel to the clivus may also be helpful for better definition of the brain-stem area. Direct coronal images may provide better definition of the temporal lobes. Ten millimeter thick sections are routinely obtained, although thinner sections (5 mm, 3 mm, 1.5 mm) are often used for better definition of the posterior fossa and brain stem. The thin sections can be reformatted as necessary. However, all artifacts seen on the actual images, such as the interpetrous artifact, will be faithfully reproduced on the reformatted images and should not be mistaken for pathology.

Brain images, both without and with intravenous contrast, are included in this chapter. Each page has been organized with the noncontrast image at the top and the contrast image at the bottom. Unlike the other chapters of the neuroradiologic portion of this atlas, the brain sections do not represent serial sections of a single individual. Instead, sections from multiple individuals were selected to demonstrate specific anatomic structures. The images have been arranged to simulate serial scans of a single patient, each series consisting of 20 images with thinner sections through the base, as indicated on the "scout view" at the beginning of each section. The noncontrast images were selected to demonstrate sulci, fissures, cisterns, and the ventricular system, as well as gray-white differentiation. The contrast scans were chosen primarily to demonstrate vascular anatomy, sometimes at the expense of other anatomic details.

Serial bone window images through the base of the skull have been included to emphasize the anatomy of the basal foramina. The fine detail of specific areas is included in the high-resolution sections of this atlas, including the temporal bone, paranasal sinuses, sella, and orbits.

A limited water-soluble contrast cisternogram is presented for more accurate demonstration of the basilar cisterns. The window settings were adjusted to provide maximum detail in the contrast-filled cisternal areas rather than in the brain parenchyma.

Brain, without and with Intravenous Contrast

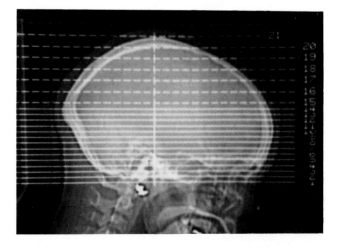

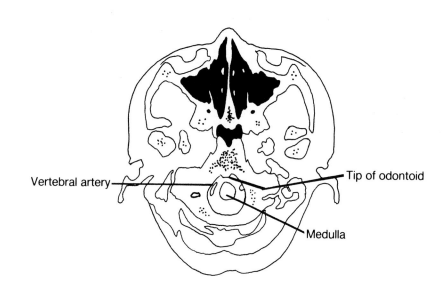

Vertebral artery — Tip of odontoid

Medulla

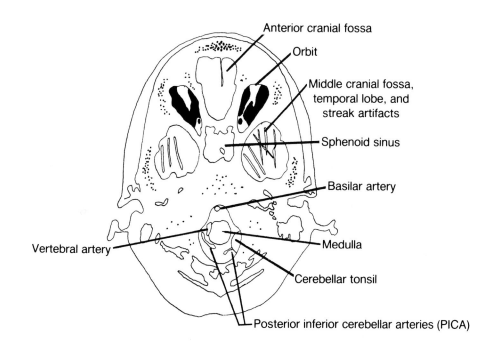

Anterior cranial fossa

Orbit

Middle cranial fossa, temporal lobe, and streak artifacts

Sphenoid sinus

Basilar artery

Vertebral artery — Medulla

Cerebellar tonsil

Posterior inferior cerebellar arteries (PICA)

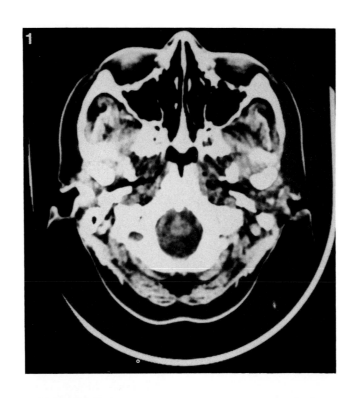

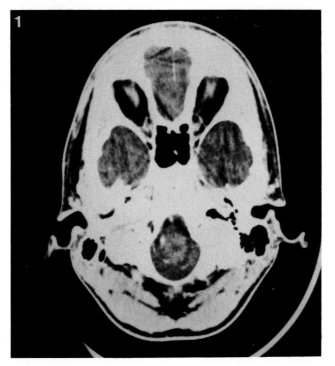

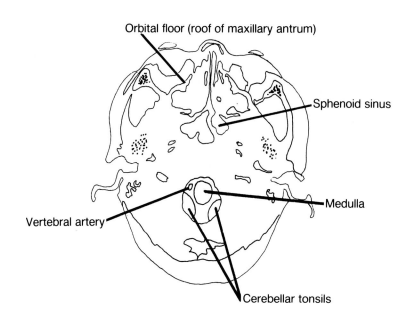

Orbital floor (roof of maxillary antrum)

Sphenoid sinus

Medulla

Vertebral artery

Cerebellar tonsils

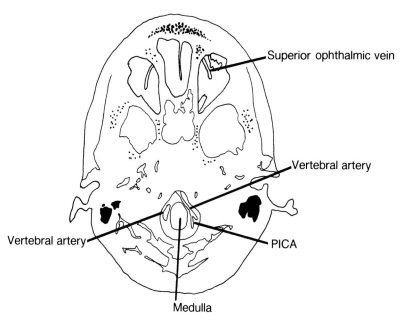

Superior ophthalmic vein

Vertebral artery

Vertebral artery

PICA

Medulla

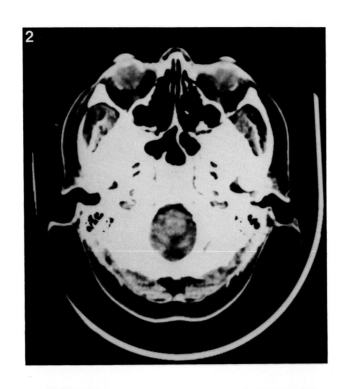

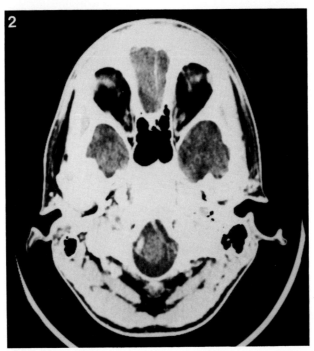

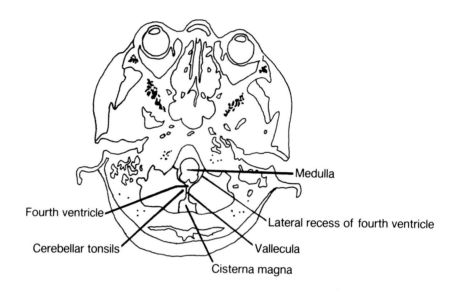

Fourth ventricle

Cerebellar tonsils

Medulla

Lateral recess of fourth ventricle

Vallecula

Cisterna magna

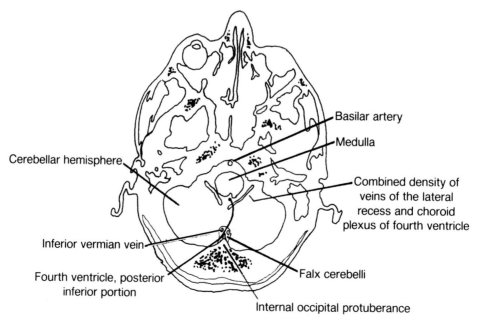

Cerebellar hemisphere

Basilar artery

Medulla

Combined density of veins of the lateral recess and choroid plexus of fourth ventricle

Inferior vermian vein

Fourth ventricle, posterior inferior portion

Falx cerebelli

Internal occipital protuberance

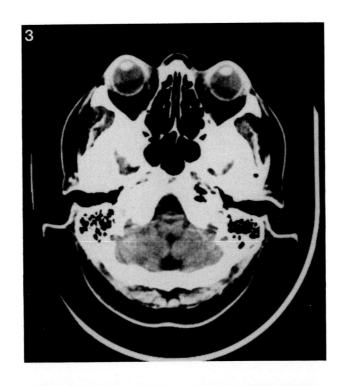

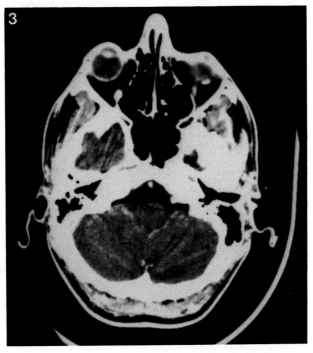

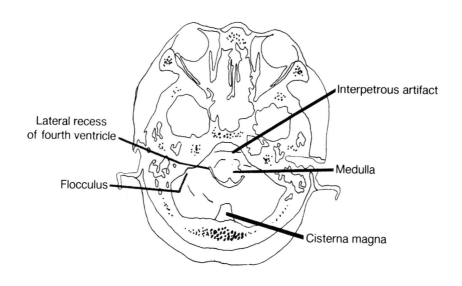

Lateral recess
of fourth ventricle

Flocculus

Interpetrous artifact

Medulla

Cisterna magna

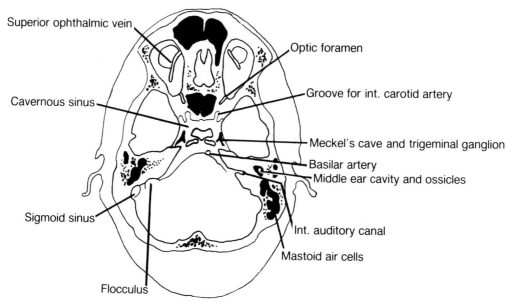

Superior ophthalmic vein

Cavernous sinus

Sigmoid sinus

Flocculus

Optic foramen

Groove for int. carotid artery

Meckel's cave and trigeminal ganglion

Basilar artery

Middle ear cavity and ossicles

Int. auditory canal

Mastoid air cells

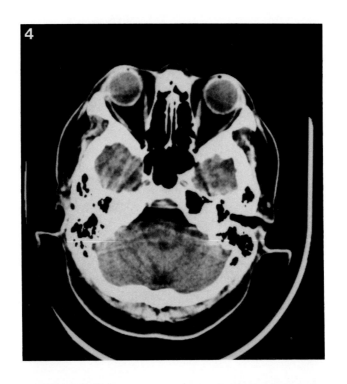

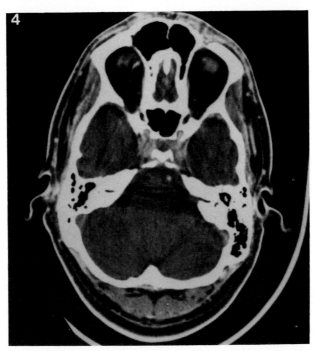

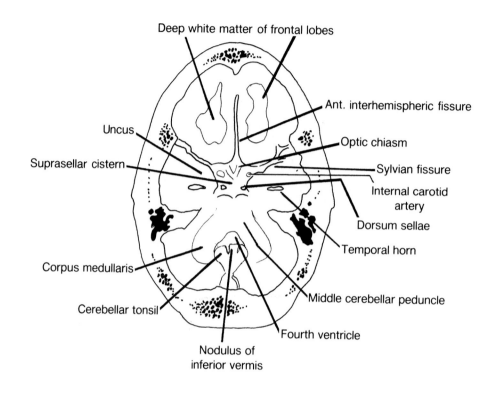

Deep white matter of frontal lobes

Ant. interhemispheric fissure

Uncus

Optic chiasm

Suprasellar cistern

Sylvian fissure

Internal carotid artery

Dorsum sellae

Temporal horn

Corpus medullaris

Cerebellar tonsil

Middle cerebellar peduncle

Fourth ventricle

Nodulus of inferior vermis

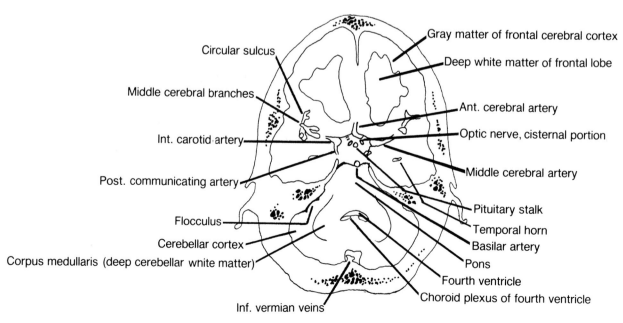

Circular sulcus

Gray matter of frontal cerebral cortex

Deep white matter of frontal lobe

Middle cerebral branches

Ant. cerebral artery

Optic nerve, cisternal portion

Int. carotid artery

Middle cerebral artery

Post. communicating artery

Pituitary stalk

Flocculus

Temporal horn

Cerebellar cortex

Basilar artery

Corpus medullaris (deep cerebellar white matter)

Pons

Fourth ventricle

Choroid plexus of fourth ventricle

Inf. vermian veins

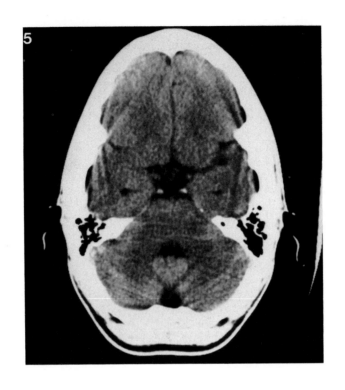

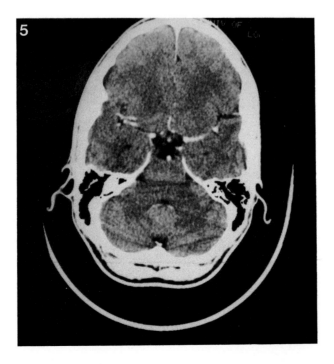

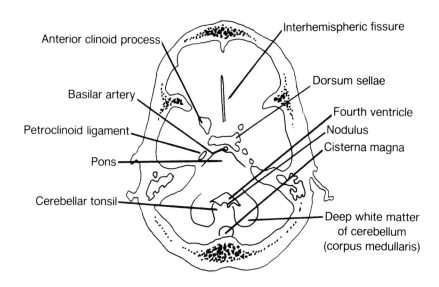

Anterior clinoid process

Basilar artery

Petroclinoid ligament

Pons

Cerebellar tonsil

Interhemispheric fissure

Dorsum sellae

Fourth ventricle

Nodulus

Cisterna magna

Deep white matter
of cerebellum
(corpus medullaris)

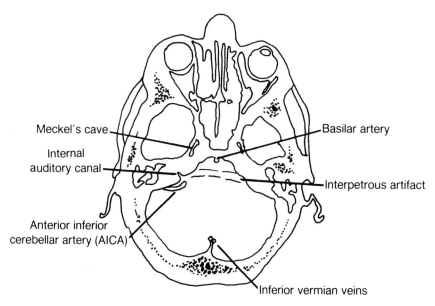

Meckel's cave

Internal
auditory canal

Anterior inferior
cerebellar artery (AICA)

Basilar artery

Interpetrous artifact

Inferior vermian veins

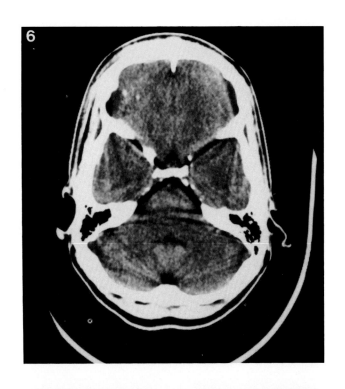

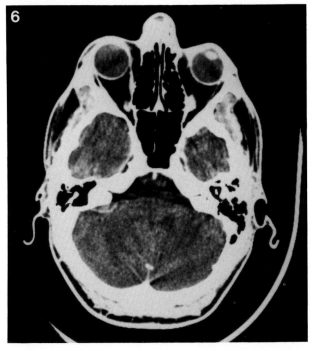

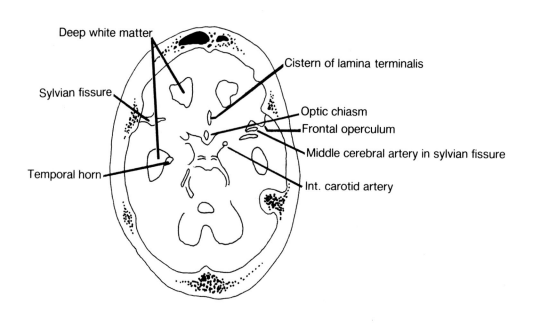

Deep white matter

Sylvian fissure

Temporal horn

Cistern of lamina terminalis

Optic chiasm

Frontal operculum

Middle cerebral artery in sylvian fissure

Int. carotid artery

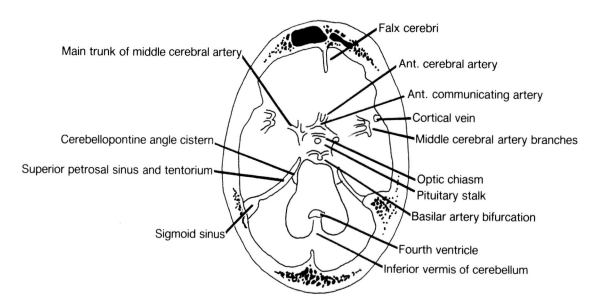

Main trunk of middle cerebral artery

Cerebellopontine angle cistern

Superior petrosal sinus and tentorium

Sigmoid sinus

Falx cerebri

Ant. cerebral artery

Ant. communicating artery

Cortical vein

Middle cerebral artery branches

Optic chiasm

Pituitary stalk

Basilar artery bifurcation

Fourth ventricle

Inferior vermis of cerebellum

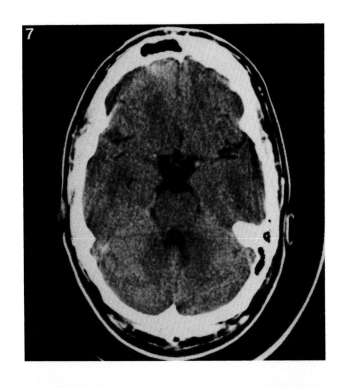

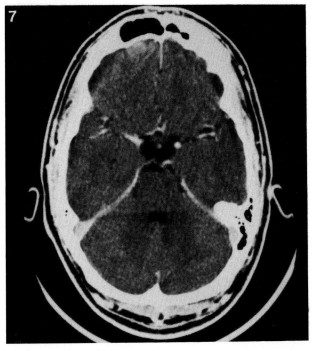

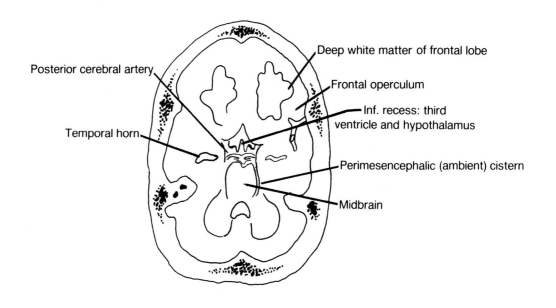

Posterior cerebral artery

Temporal horn

Deep white matter of frontal lobe

Frontal operculum

Inf. recess: third ventricle and hypothalamus

Perimesencephalic (ambient) cistern

Midbrain

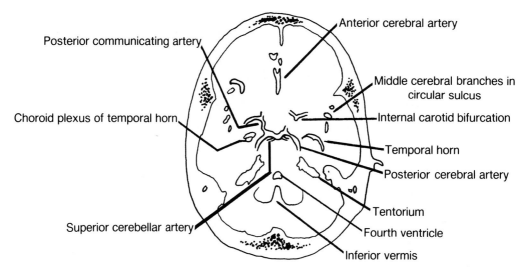

Posterior communicating artery

Choroid plexus of temporal horn

Superior cerebellar artery

Anterior cerebral artery

Middle cerebral branches in circular sulcus

Internal carotid bifurcation

Temporal horn

Posterior cerebral artery

Tentorium

Fourth ventricle

Inferior vermis

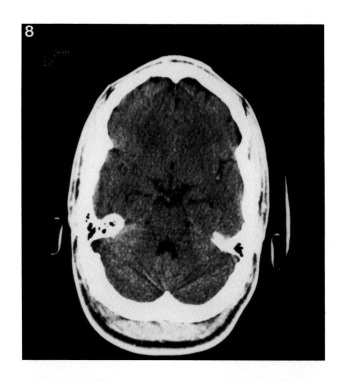

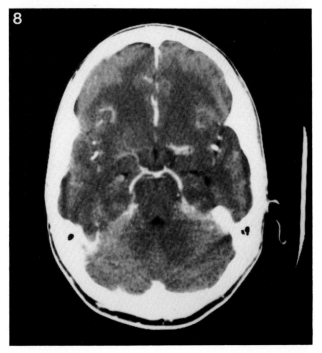

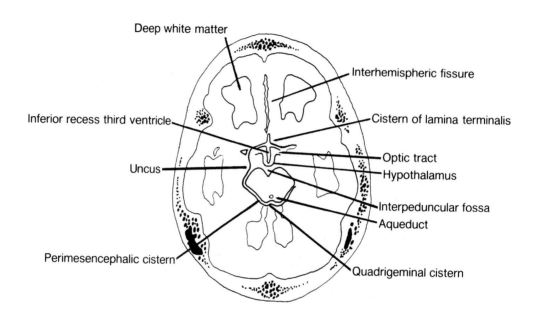

Deep white matter

Interhemispheric fissure

Inferior recess third ventricle

Cistern of lamina terminalis

Optic tract

Uncus

Hypothalamus

Interpeduncular fossa

Aqueduct

Perimesencephalic cistern

Quadrigeminal cistern

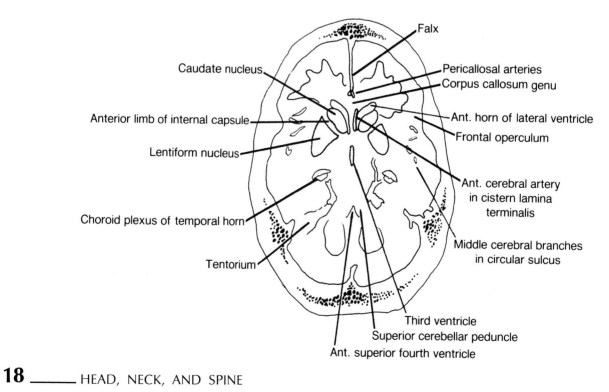

Falx

Caudate nucleus

Pericallosal arteries

Corpus callosum genu

Anterior limb of internal capsule

Ant. horn of lateral ventricle

Frontal operculum

Lentiform nucleus

Ant. cerebral artery
in cistern lamina
terminalis

Choroid plexus of temporal horn

Middle cerebral branches
in circular sulcus

Tentorium

Third ventricle

Superior cerebellar peduncle

Ant. superior fourth ventricle

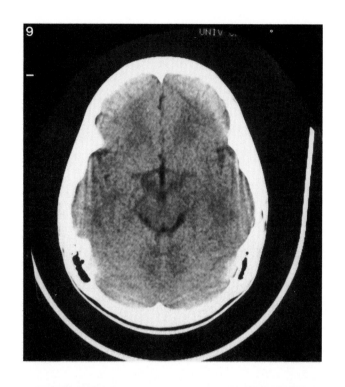

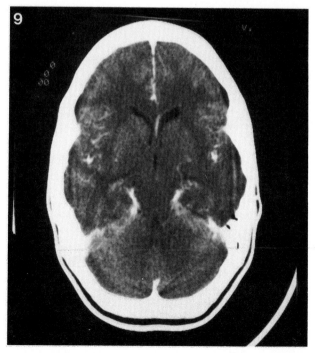

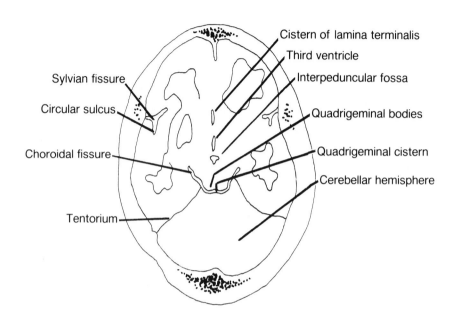

Cistern of lamina terminalis

Third ventricle

Interpeduncular fossa

Sylvian fissure

Circular sulcus

Quadrigeminal bodies

Choroidal fissure

Quadrigeminal cistern

Cerebellar hemisphere

Tentorium

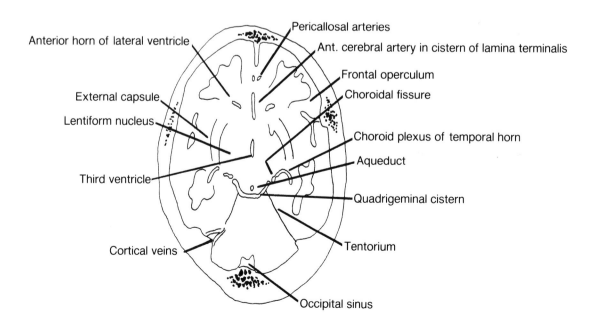

Pericallosal arteries

Anterior horn of lateral ventricle

Ant. cerebral artery in cistern of lamina terminalis

Frontal operculum

External capsule

Choroidal fissure

Lentiform nucleus

Choroid plexus of temporal horn

Aqueduct

Third ventricle

Quadrigeminal cistern

Cortical veins

Tentorium

Occipital sinus

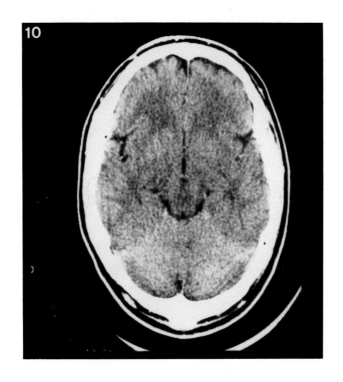

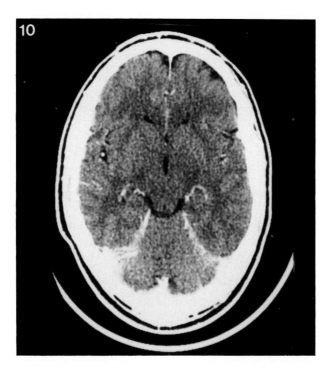

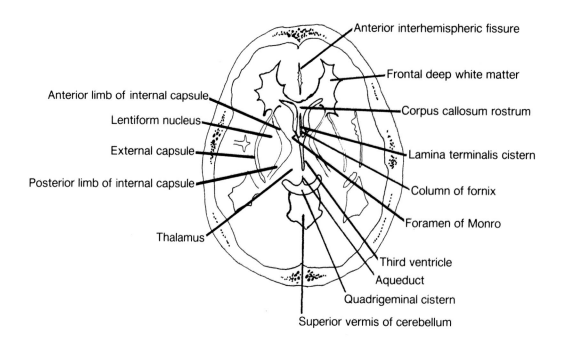

Anterior interhemispheric fissure

Frontal deep white matter

Corpus callosum rostrum

Lamina terminalis cistern

Column of fornix

Foramen of Monro

Third ventricle

Aqueduct

Quadrigeminal cistern

Superior vermis of cerebellum

Anterior limb of internal capsule

Lentiform nucleus

External capsule

Posterior limb of internal capsule

Thalamus

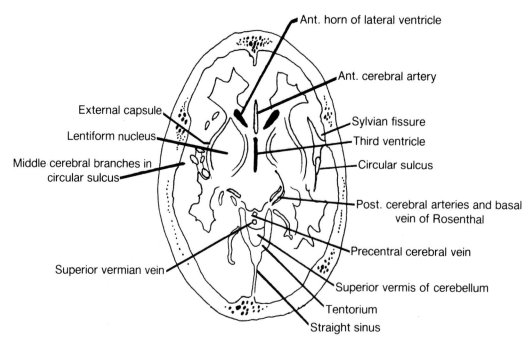

Ant. horn of lateral ventricle

Ant. cerebral artery

Sylvian fissure

Third ventricle

Circular sulcus

Post. cerebral arteries and basal vein of Rosenthal

Precentral cerebral vein

Superior vermis of cerebellum

Tentorium

Straight sinus

External capsule

Lentiform nucleus

Middle cerebral branches in circular sulcus

Superior vermian vein

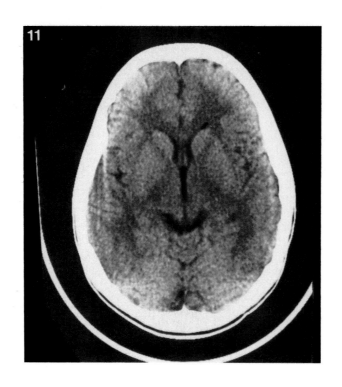

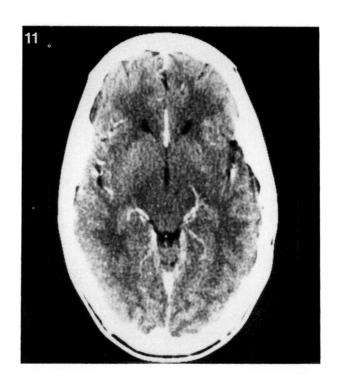

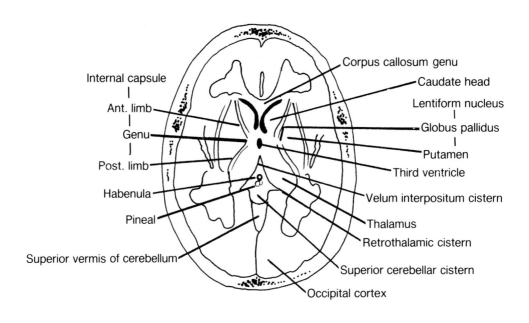

Internal capsule

Ant. limb

Genu

Post. limb

Habenula

Pineal

Superior vermis of cerebellum

Corpus callosum genu

Caudate head

Lentiform nucleus

Globus pallidus

Putamen

Third ventricle

Velum interpositum cistern

Thalamus

Retrothalamic cistern

Superior cerebellar cistern

Occipital cortex

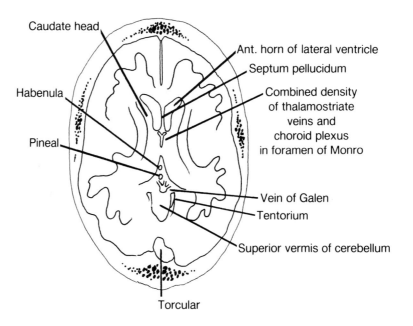

Caudate head

Habenula

Pineal

Ant. horn of lateral ventricle

Septum pellucidum

Combined density
of thalamostriate
veins and
choroid plexus
in foramen of Monro

Vein of Galen

Tentorium

Superior vermis of cerebellum

Torcular

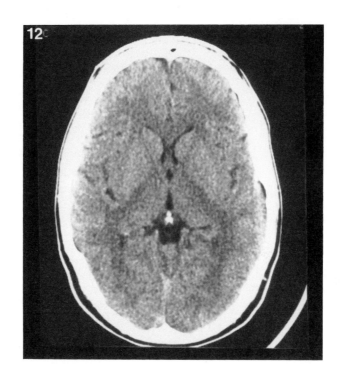

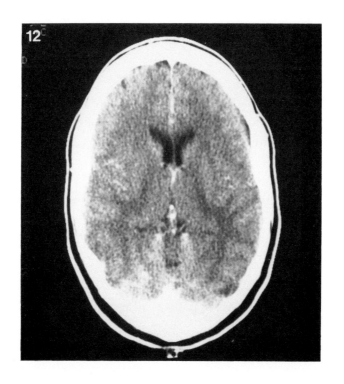

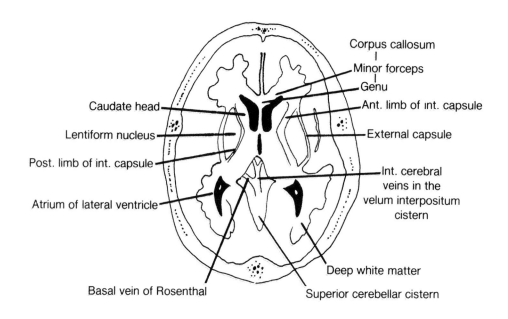

Corpus callosum

Minor forceps

Genu

Caudate head

Ant. limb of int. capsule

Lentiform nucleus

External capsule

Post. limb of int. capsule

Int. cerebral veins in the velum interpositum cistern

Atrium of lateral ventricle

Deep white matter

Basal vein of Rosenthal

Superior cerebellar cistern

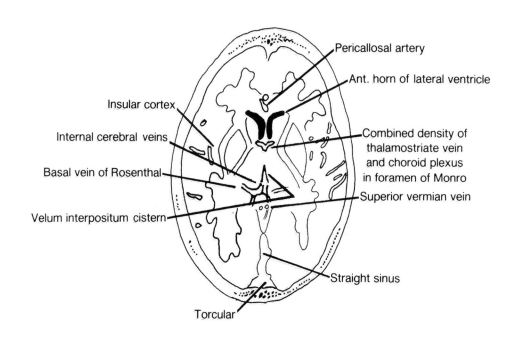

Pericallosal artery

Ant. horn of lateral ventricle

Insular cortex

Internal cerebral veins

Combined density of thalamostriate vein and choroid plexus in foramen of Monro

Basal vein of Rosenthal

Superior vermian vein

Velum interpositum cistern

Straight sinus

Torcular

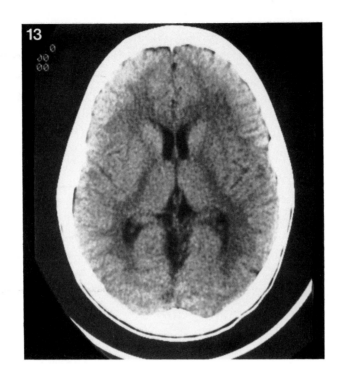

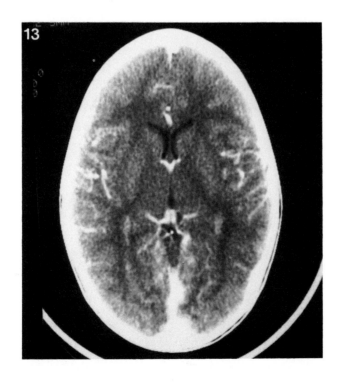

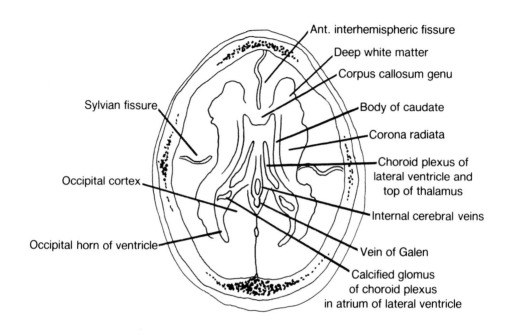

Ant. interhemispheric fissure

Deep white matter

Corpus callosum genu

Body of caudate

Corona radiata

Choroid plexus of
lateral ventricle and
top of thalamus

Internal cerebral veins

Vein of Galen

Calcified glomus
of choroid plexus
in atrium of lateral ventricle

Sylvian fissure

Occipital cortex

Occipital horn of ventricle

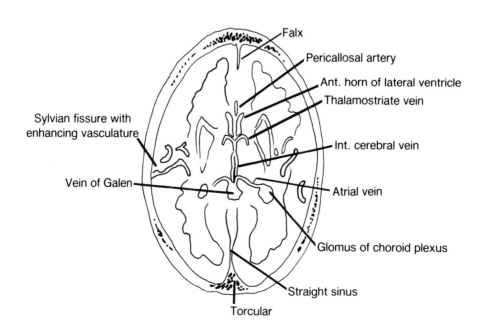

Falx

Pericallosal artery

Ant. horn of lateral ventricle

Thalamostriate vein

Int. cerebral vein

Atrial vein

Glomus of choroid plexus

Straight sinus

Torcular

Sylvian fissure with
enhancing vasculature

Vein of Galen

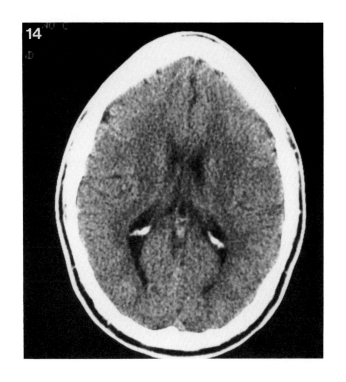

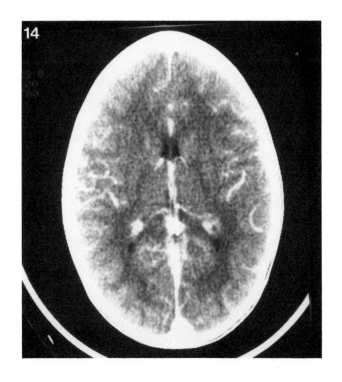

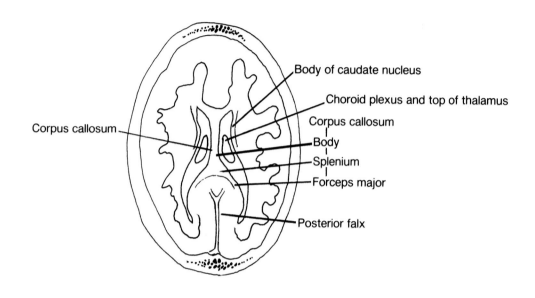

Corpus callosum

Body of caudate nucleus

Choroid plexus and top of thalamus

Corpus callosum

Body

Splenium

Forceps major

Posterior falx

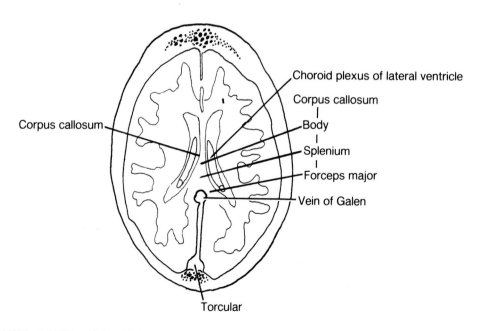

Corpus callosum

Choroid plexus of lateral ventricle

Corpus callosum

Body

Splenium

Forceps major

Vein of Galen

Torcular

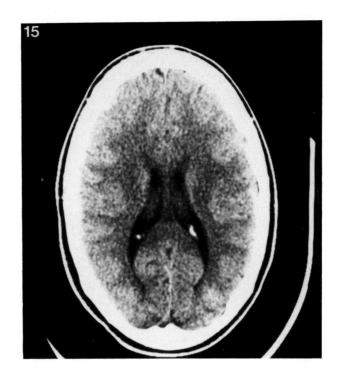

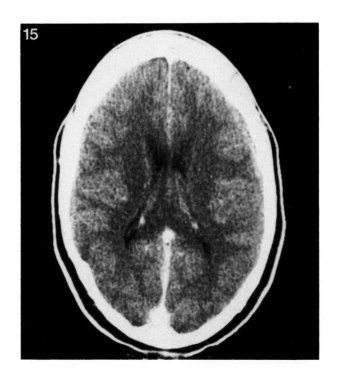

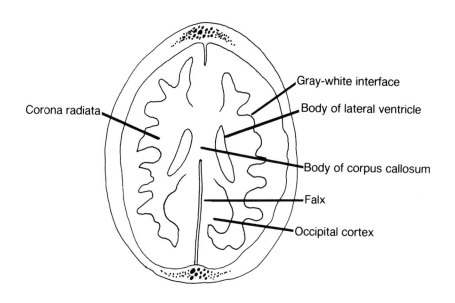

Corona radiata

Gray-white interface

Body of lateral ventricle

Body of corpus callosum

Falx

Occipital cortex

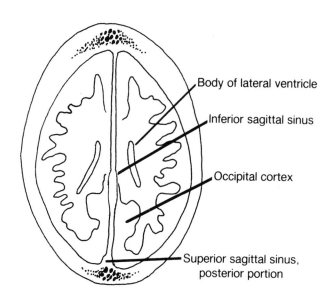

Body of lateral ventricle

Inferior sagittal sinus

Occipital cortex

Superior sagittal sinus, posterior portion

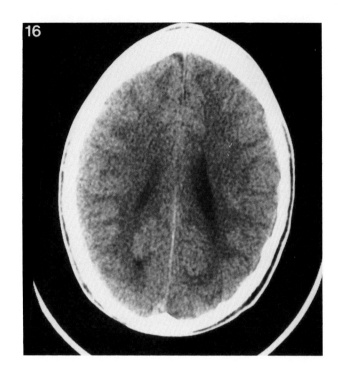

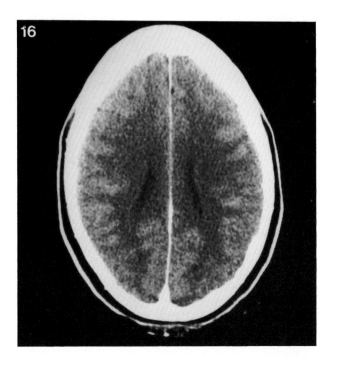

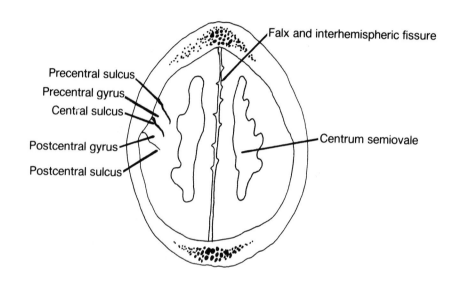

Falx and interhemispheric fissure

Precentral sulcus

Precentral gyrus

Central sulcus

Postcentral gyrus

Postcentral sulcus

Centrum semiovale

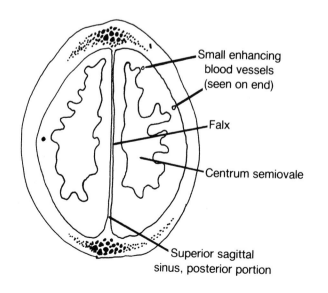

Small enhancing
blood vessels
(seen on end)

Falx

Centrum semiovale

Superior sagittal
sinus, posterior portion

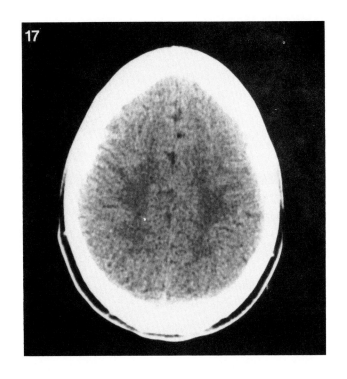

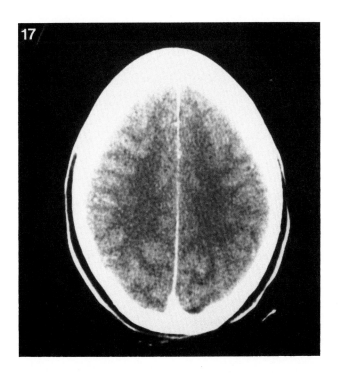

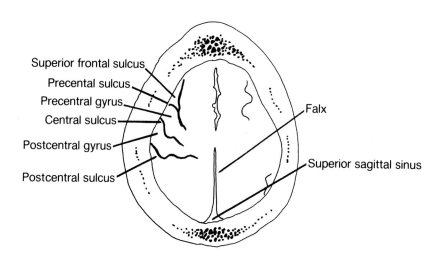

Superior frontal sulcus

Precental sulcus

Precentral gyrus

Central sulcus

Postcentral gyrus

Postcentral sulcus

Falx

Superior sagittal sinus

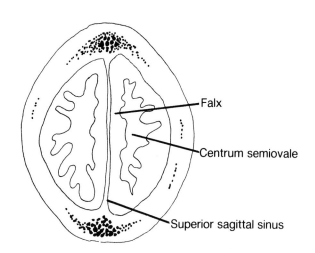

Falx

Centrum semiovale

Superior sagittal sinus

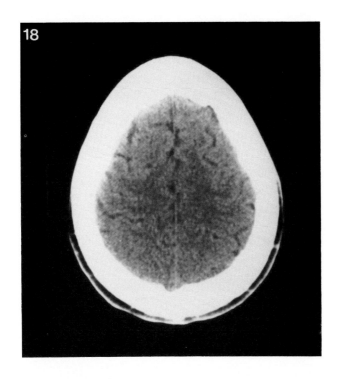

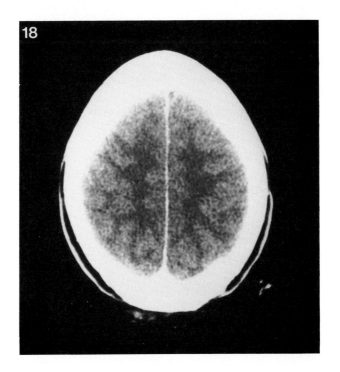

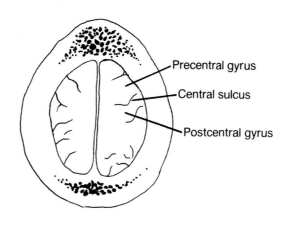

Precentral gyrus

Central sulcus

Postcentral gyrus

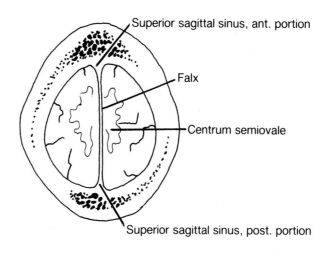

Superior sagittal sinus, ant. portion

Falx

Centrum semiovale

Superior sagittal sinus, post. portion

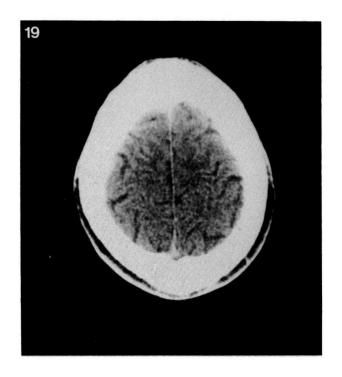

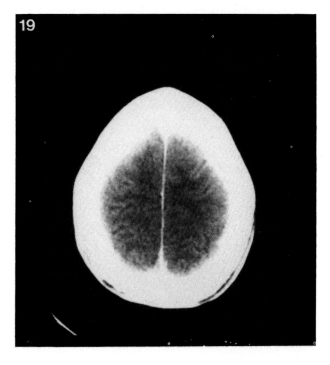

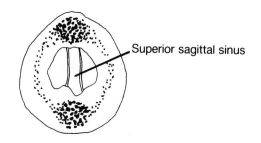

Superior sagittal sinus

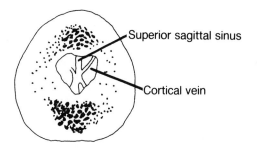

Superior sagittal sinus

Cortical vein

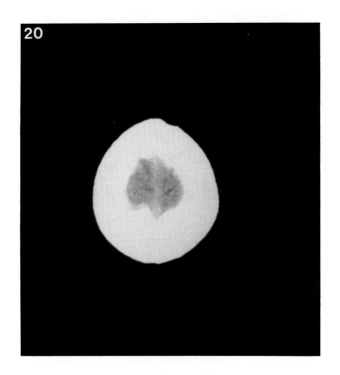

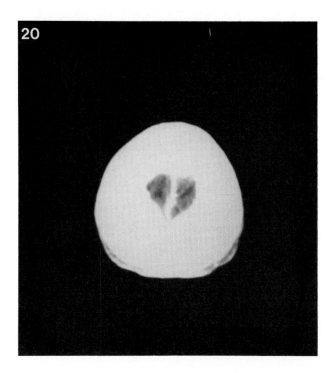

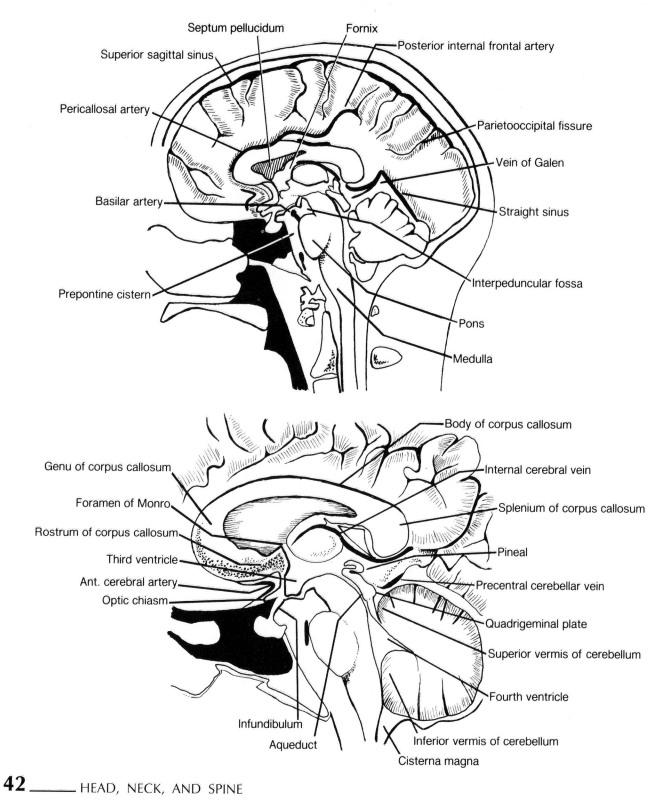

Septum pellucidum

Fornix

Superior sagittal sinus

Posterior internal frontal artery

Pericallosal artery

Parietooccipital fissure

Vein of Galen

Basilar artery

Straight sinus

Interpeduncular fossa

Prepontine cistern

Pons

Medulla

Body of corpus callosum

Genu of corpus callosum

Internal cerebral vein

Foramen of Monro

Splenium of corpus callosum

Rostrum of corpus callosum

Third ventricle

Pineal

Ant. cerebral artery

Precentral cerebellar vein

Optic chiasm

Quadrigeminal plate

Superior vermis of cerebellum

Fourth ventricle

Infundibulum

Inferior vermis of cerebellum

Aqueduct

Cisterna magna

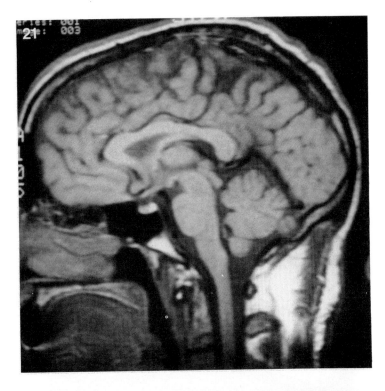

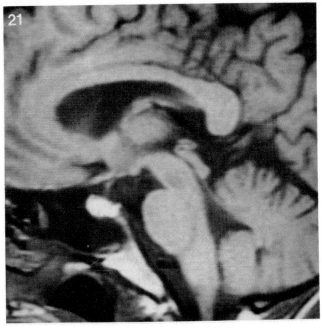

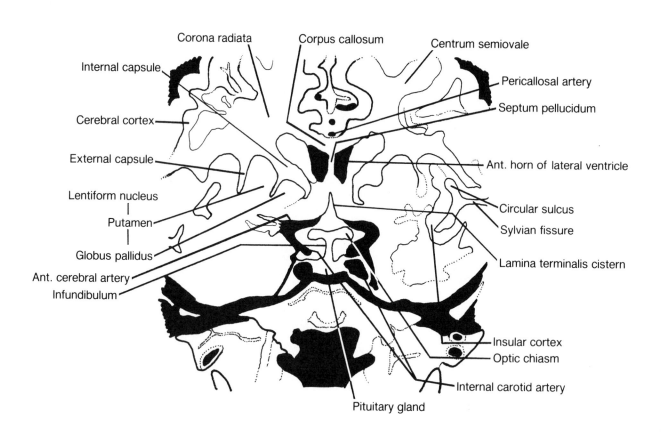

Corona radiata

Corpus callosum

Centrum semiovale

Internal capsule

Pericallosal artery

Septum pellucidum

Cerebral cortex

External capsule

Ant. horn of lateral ventricle

Lentiform nucleus

Circular sulcus

Putamen

Sylvian fissure

Globus pallidus

Lamina terminalis cistern

Ant. cerebral artery

Infundibulum

Insular cortex

Optic chiasm

Internal carotid artery

Pituitary gland

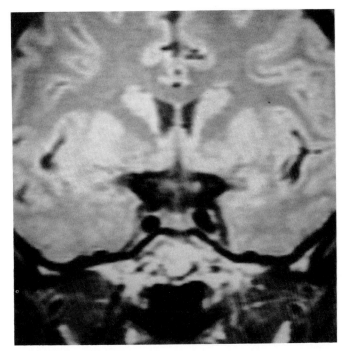

Coronal MRI of the brain at the level of the sella turcica.

Skull Base

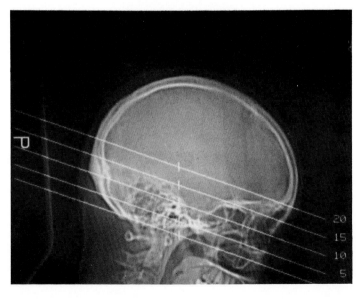

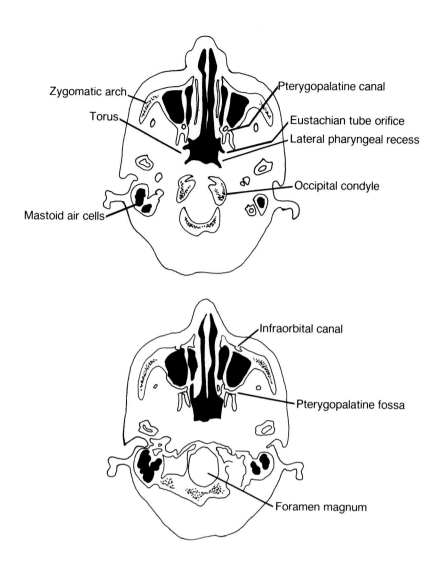

Zygomatic arch

Torus

Mastoid air cells

Pterygopalatine canal

Eustachian tube orifice

Lateral pharyngeal recess

Occipital condyle

Infraorbital canal

Pterygopalatine fossa

Foramen magnum

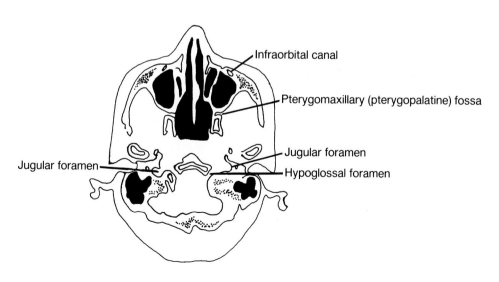

Infraorbital canal

Pterygomaxillary (pterygopalatine) fossa

Jugular foramen

Jugular foramen

Hypoglossal foramen

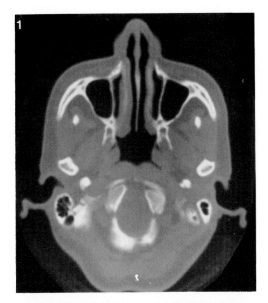

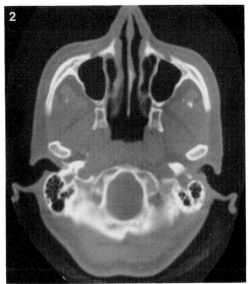

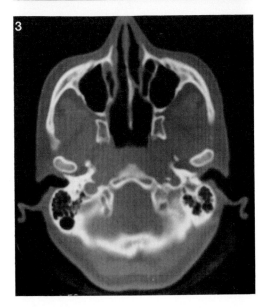

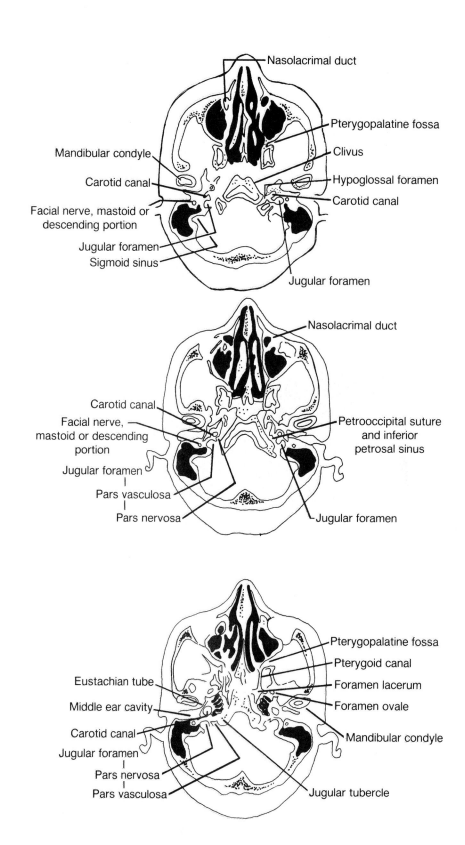

Nasolacrimal duct

Pterygopalatine fossa

Clivus

Hypoglossal foramen

Carotid canal

Mandibular condyle

Carotid canal

Facial nerve, mastoid or descending portion

Jugular foramen

Sigmoid sinus

Jugular foramen

Nasolacrimal duct

Carotid canal

Facial nerve, mastoid or descending portion

Petrooccipital suture and inferior petrosal sinus

Jugular foramen

Pars vasculosa

Pars nervosa

Jugular foramen

Pterygopalatine fossa

Pterygoid canal

Foramen lacerum

Foramen ovale

Mandibular condyle

Jugular tubercle

Eustachian tube

Middle ear cavity

Carotid canal

Jugular foramen

Pars nervosa

Pars vasculosa

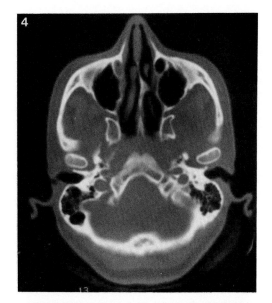

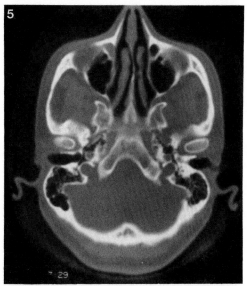

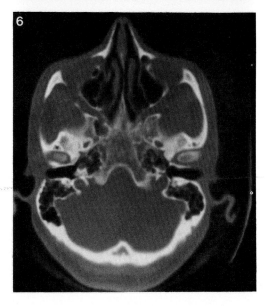

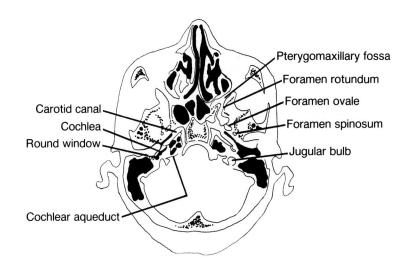

Carotid canal

Cochlea

Round window

Cochlear aqueduct

Pterygomaxillary fossa

Foramen rotundum

Foramen ovale

Foramen spinosum

Jugular bulb

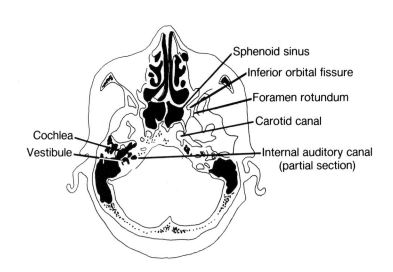

Cochlea

Vestibule

Sphenoid sinus

Inferior orbital fissure

Foramen rotundum

Carotid canal

Internal auditory canal
(partial section)

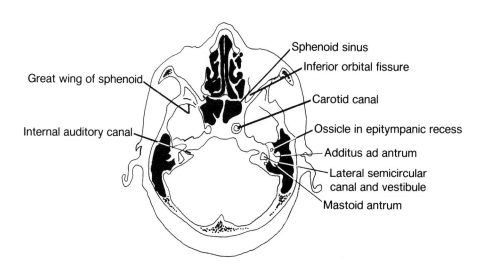

Great wing of sphenoid

Internal auditory canal

Sphenoid sinus

Inferior orbital fissure

Carotid canal

Ossicle in epitympanic recess

Additus ad antrum

Lateral semicircular
canal and vestibule

Mastoid antrum

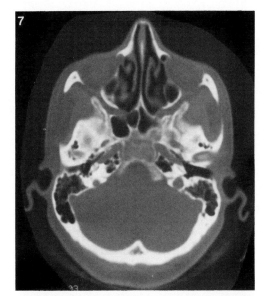

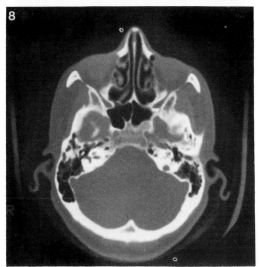

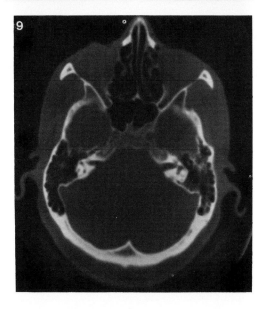

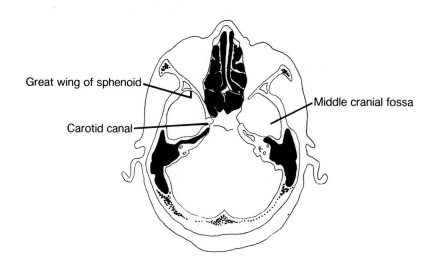

Great wing of sphenoid

Carotid canal

Middle cranial fossa

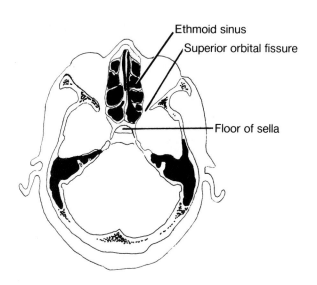

Ethmoid sinus

Superior orbital fissure

Floor of sella

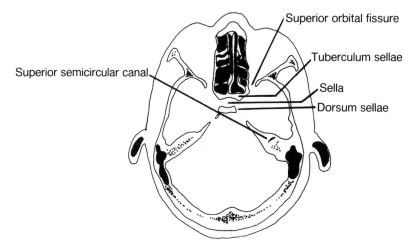

Superior orbital fissure

Tuberculum sellae

Sella

Dorsum sellae

Superior semicircular canal

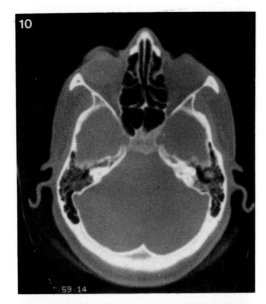

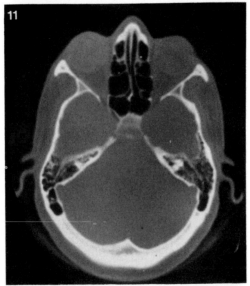

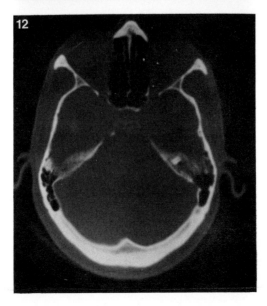

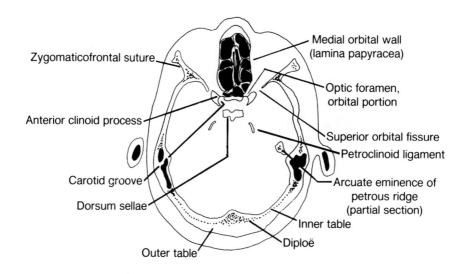

Zygomaticofrontal suture

Anterior clinoid process

Carotid groove

Dorsum sellae

Medial orbital wall
(lamina papyracea)

Optic foramen,
orbital portion

Superior orbital fissure

Petroclinoid ligament

Arcuate eminence of
petrous ridge
(partial section)

Inner table

Diploë

Outer table

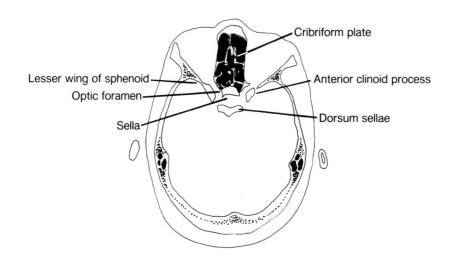

Cribriform plate

Lesser wing of sphenoid

Optic foramen

Sella

Anterior clinoid process

Dorsum sellae

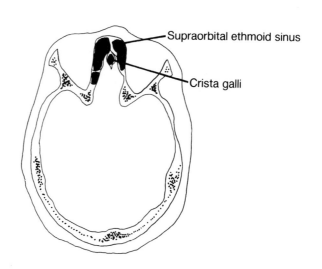

Supraorbital ethmoid sinus

Crista galli

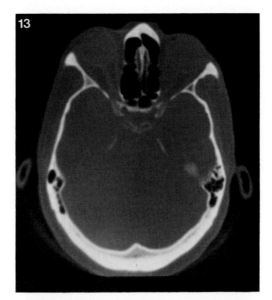

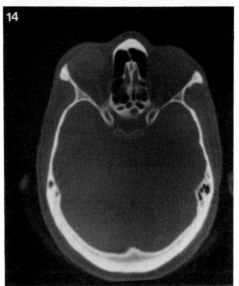

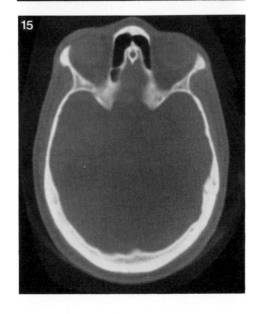

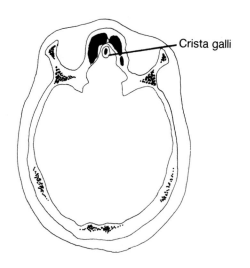

Crista galli

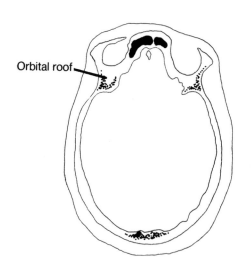

Orbital roof

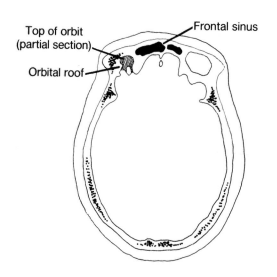

Top of orbit
(partial section)

Frontal sinus

Orbital roof

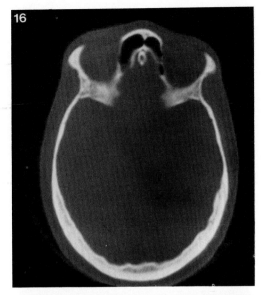

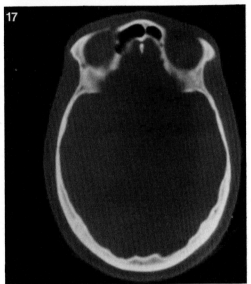

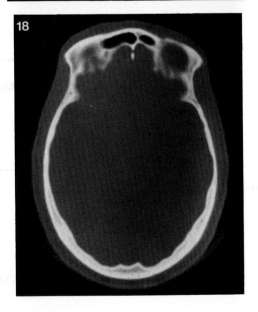

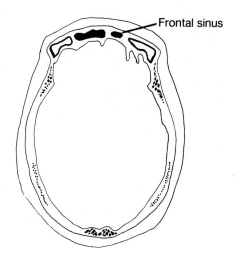

Frontal sinus

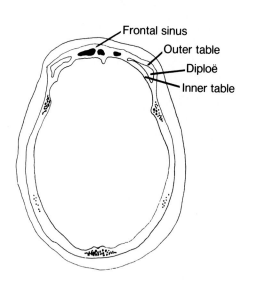

Frontal sinus

Outer table

Diploë

Inner table

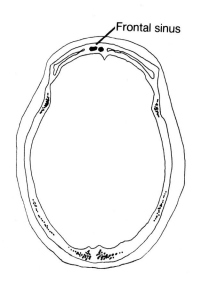

Frontal sinus

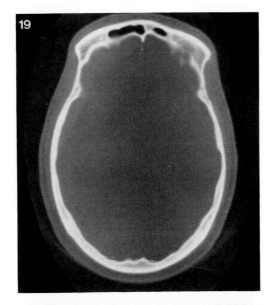

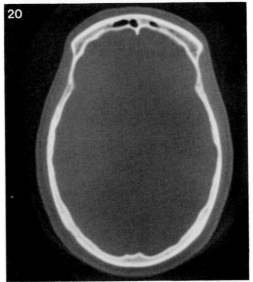

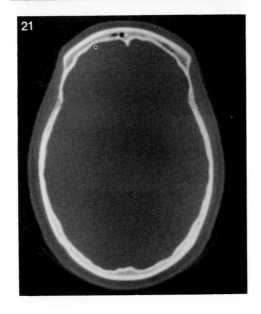

Cisternogram: Axial

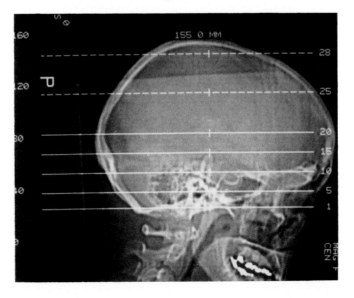

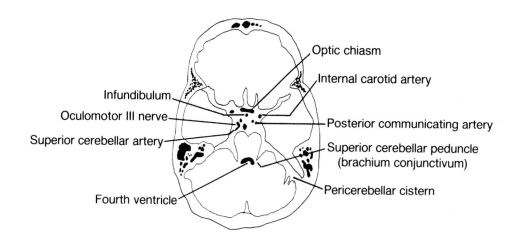

Optic chiasm

Internal carotid artery

Infundibulum

Oculomotor III nerve

Posterior communicating artery

Superior cerebellar artery

Superior cerebellar peduncle
(brachium conjunctivum)

Pericerebellar cistern

Fourth ventricle

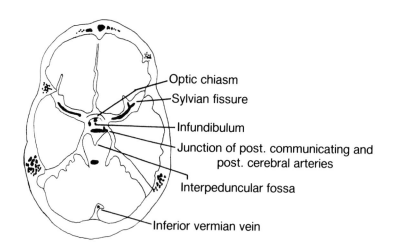

Optic chiasm

Sylvian fissure

Infundibulum

Junction of post. communicating and
post. cerebral arteries

Interpeduncular fossa

Inferior vermian vein

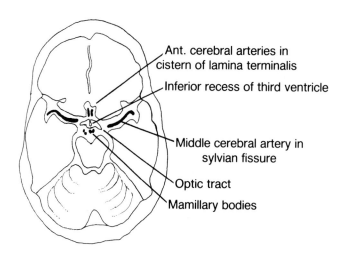

Ant. cerebral arteries in
cistern of lamina terminalis

Inferior recess of third ventricle

Middle cerebral artery in
sylvian fissure

Optic tract

Mamillary bodies

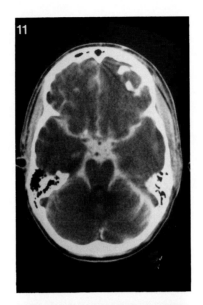

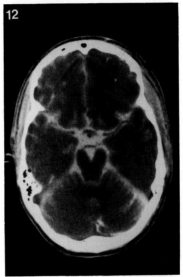

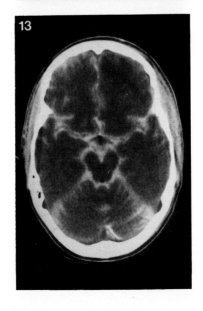

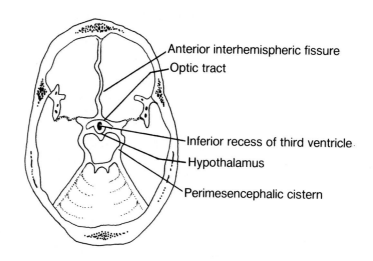

Anterior interhemispheric fissure

Optic tract

Inferior recess of third ventricle

Hypothalamus

Perimesencephalic cistern

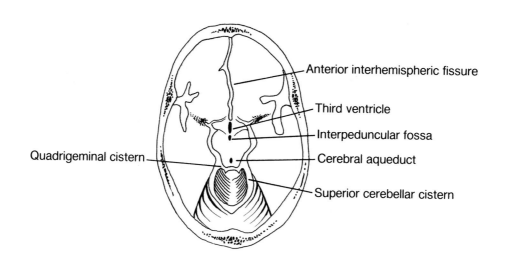

Anterior interhemispheric fissure

Third ventricle

Interpeduncular fossa

Quadrigeminal cistern

Cerebral aqueduct

Superior cerebellar cistern

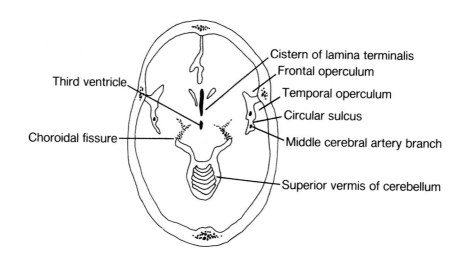

Third ventricle

Choroidal fissure

Cistern of lamina terminalis

Frontal operculum

Temporal operculum

Circular sulcus

Middle cerebral artery branch

Superior vermis of cerebellum

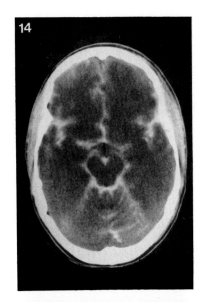

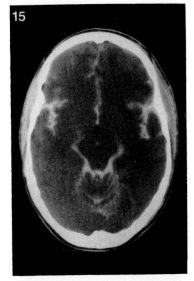

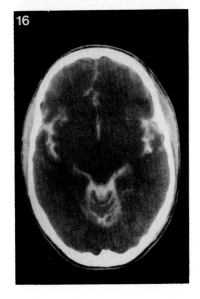

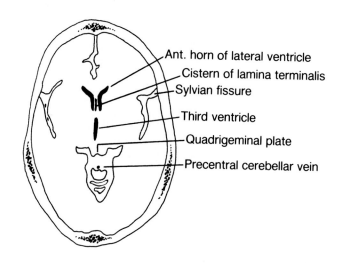

Ant. horn of lateral ventricle

Cistern of lamina terminalis

Sylvian fissure

Third ventricle

Quadrigeminal plate

Precentral cerebellar vein

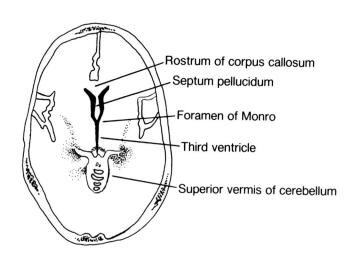

Rostrum of corpus callosum

Septum pellucidum

Foramen of Monro

Third ventricle

Superior vermis of cerebellum

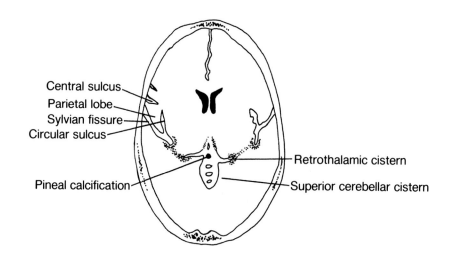

Central sulcus

Parietal lobe

Sylvian fissure

Circular sulcus

Pineal calcification

Retrothalamic cistern

Superior cerebellar cistern

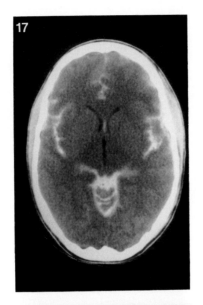

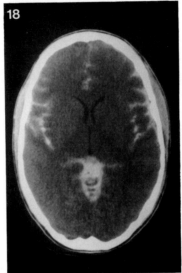

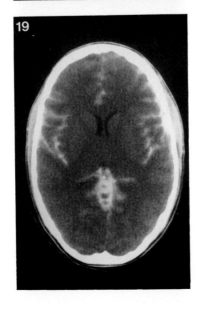

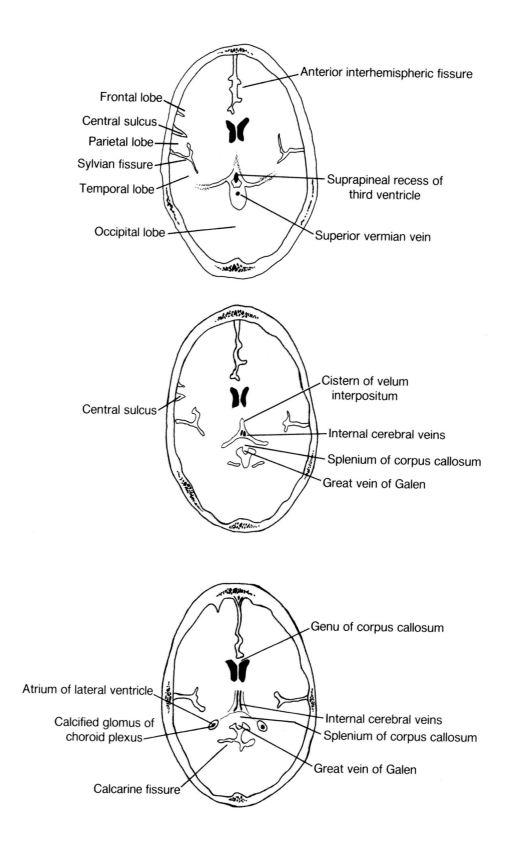

Anterior interhemispheric fissure

Frontal lobe

Central sulcus

Parietal lobe

Sylvian fissure

Temporal lobe

Suprapineal recess of third ventricle

Occipital lobe

Superior vermian vein

Central sulcus

Cistern of velum interpositum

Internal cerebral veins

Splenium of corpus callosum

Great vein of Galen

Genu of corpus callosum

Atrium of lateral ventricle

Calcified glomus of choroid plexus

Internal cerebral veins

Splenium of corpus callosum

Great vein of Galen

Calcarine fissure

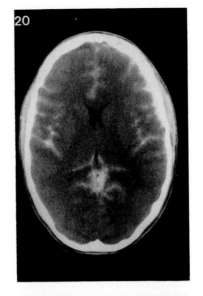

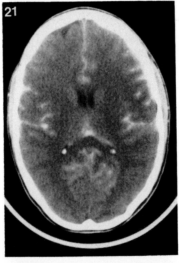

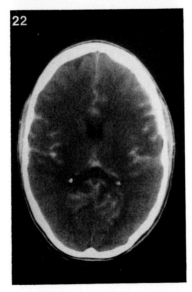

Cisternogram: Coronal

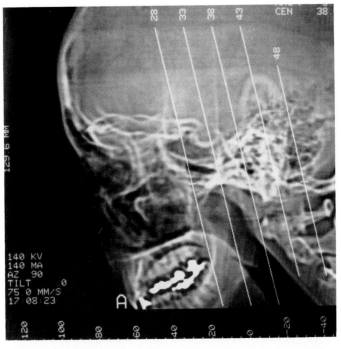

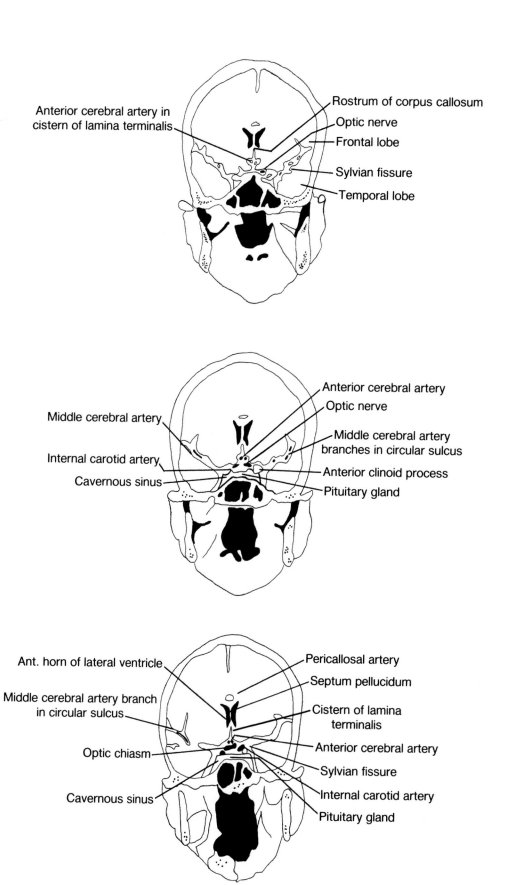

Anterior cerebral artery in cistern of lamina terminalis

Rostrum of corpus callosum

Optic nerve

Frontal lobe

Sylvian fissure

Temporal lobe

Middle cerebral artery

Anterior cerebral artery

Optic nerve

Middle cerebral artery branches in circular sulcus

Internal carotid artery

Cavernous sinus

Anterior clinoid process

Pituitary gland

Ant. horn of lateral ventricle

Pericallosal artery

Septum pellucidum

Middle cerebral artery branch in circular sulcus

Cistern of lamina terminalis

Optic chiasm

Anterior cerebral artery

Sylvian fissure

Internal carotid artery

Cavernous sinus

Pituitary gland

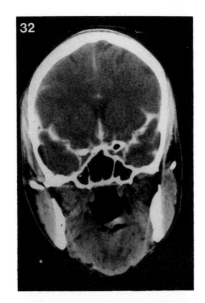

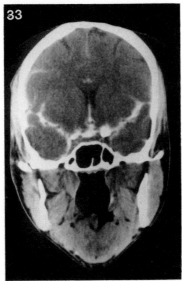

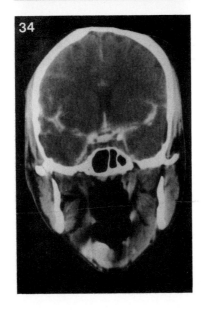

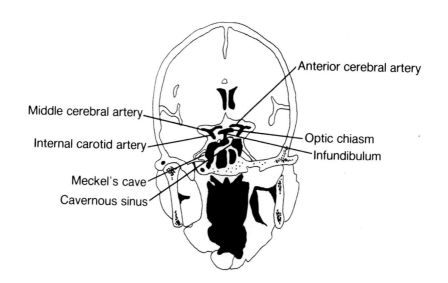

Anterior cerebral artery

Middle cerebral artery

Internal carotid artery

Meckel's cave

Cavernous sinus

Optic chiasm

Infundibulum

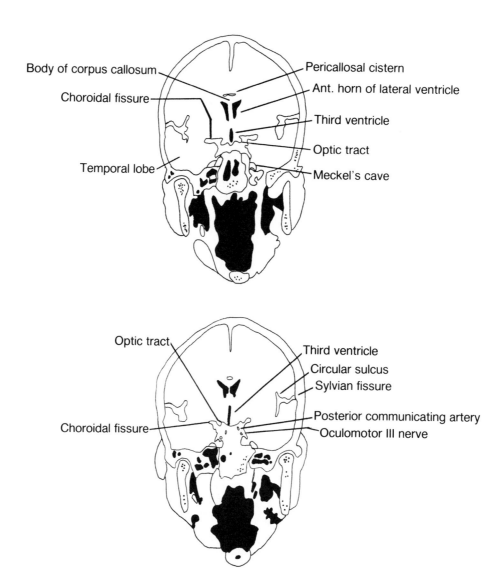

Body of corpus callosum

Choroidal fissure

Temporal lobe

Pericallosal cistern

Ant. horn of lateral ventricle

Third ventricle

Optic tract

Meckel's cave

Optic tract

Choroidal fissure

Third ventricle

Circular sulcus

Sylvian fissure

Posterior communicating artery

Oculomotor III nerve

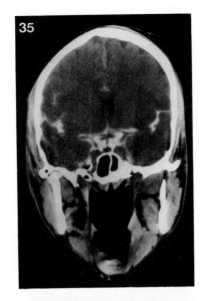

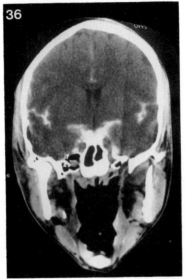

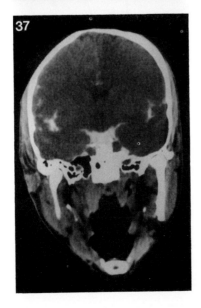

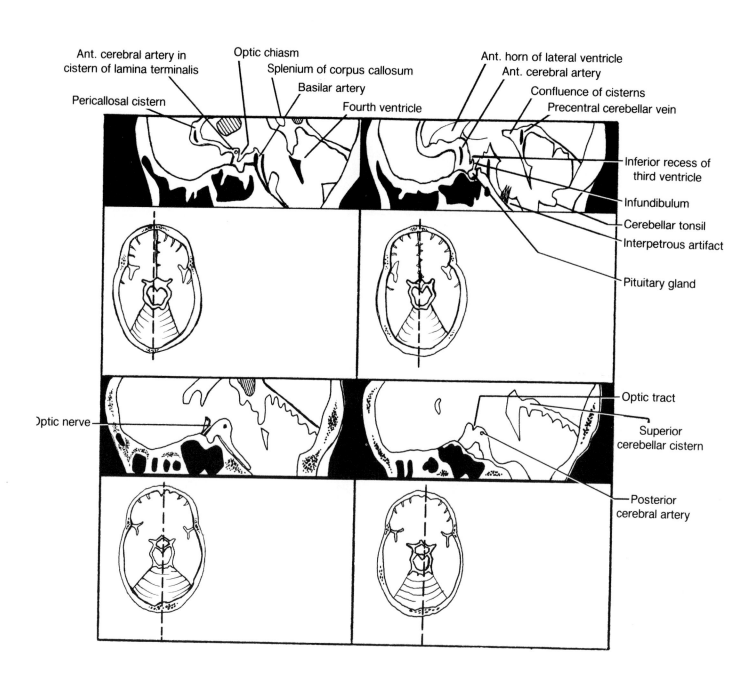

Ant. cerebral artery in cistern of lamina terminalis

Pericallosal cistern

Optic chiasm

Splenium of corpus callosum

Basilar artery

Fourth ventricle

Ant. horn of lateral ventricle

Ant. cerebral artery

Confluence of cisterns

Precentral cerebellar vein

Inferior recess of third ventricle

Infundibulum

Cerebellar tonsil

Interpetrous artifact

Pituitary gland

Optic nerve

Optic tract

Superior cerebellar cistern

Posterior cerebral artery

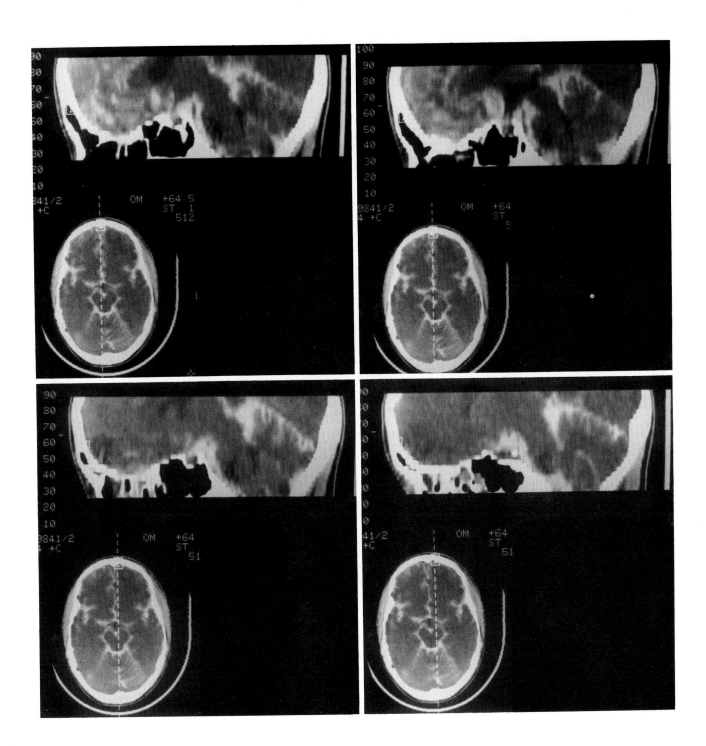

2 Sella and Juxtasella

The rapid intravenous administration of high-dose (80 gm I) contrast is usually employed. Direct coronal or axial sections of 1.5 mm thickness with reformating in sagittal or coronal planes are routinely used. All artifacts present on axial images will be reproduced on reformatted images, which may result in artifactual low densities within the sella. Dental restorations may degrade coronal images. Reformatted images may better define the pituitary stalk if coronal scan planes cannot be achieved parallel to the stalk. The availability of more rapid image acquisition and processing on contemporary scanners has decreased the time necessary to perform this protocol for pituitary stalk imaging.

Soft tissue and bone window images are provided in both axial and coronal planes, as well as reformatted images in sagittal and coronal planes.

Sella and Juxtasella with Intravenous Contrast: Axial Plane

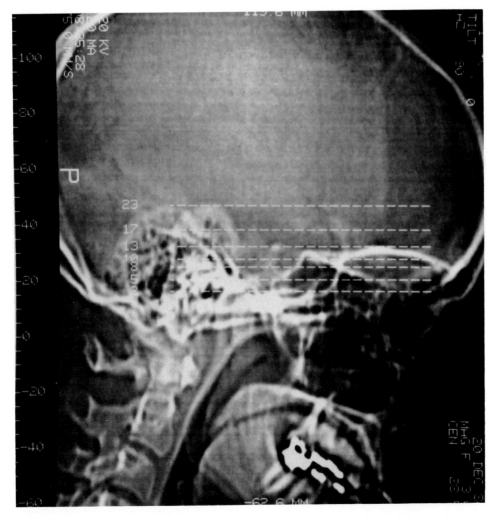

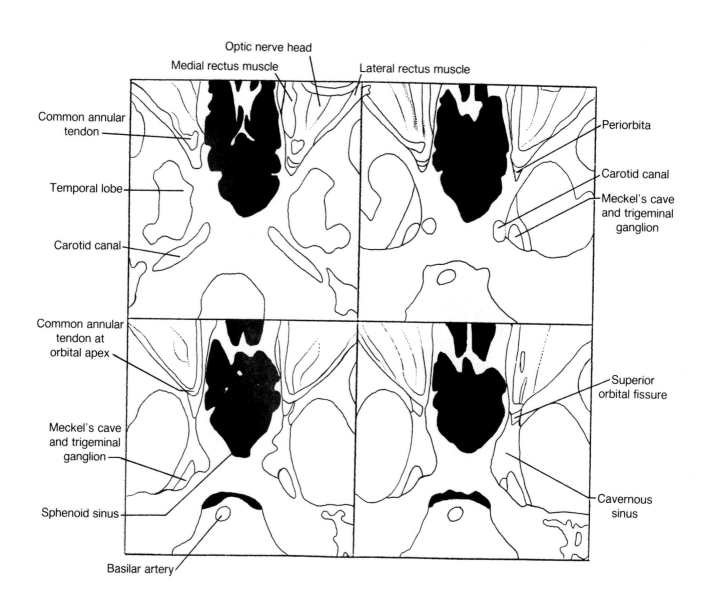

Optic nerve head

Medial rectus muscle

Lateral rectus muscle

Common annular tendon

Periorbita

Carotid canal

Meckel's cave and trigeminal ganglion

Temporal lobe

Carotid canal

Common annular tendon at orbital apex

Superior orbital fissure

Meckel's cave and trigeminal ganglion

Sphenoid sinus

Cavernous sinus

Basilar artery

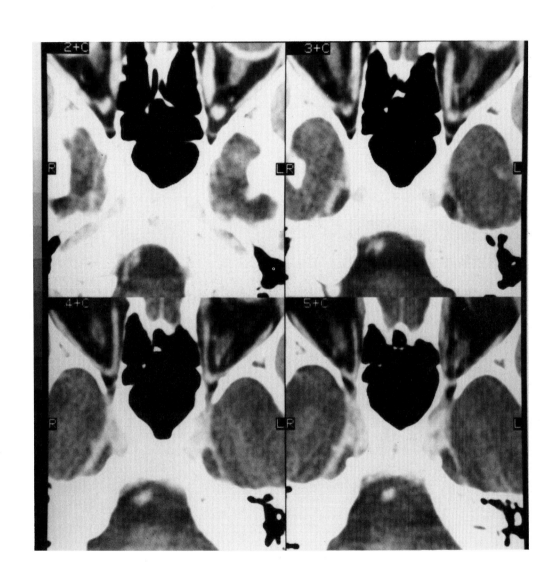

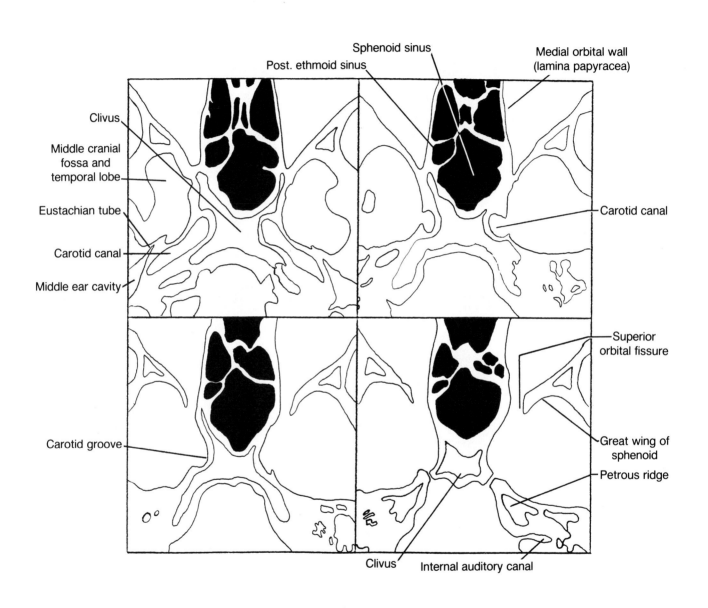

Sphenoid sinus

Post. ethmoid sinus

Medial orbital wall
(lamina papyracea)

Clivus

Middle cranial
fossa and
temporal lobe

Eustachian tube

Carotid canal

Middle ear cavity

Carotid canal

Carotid groove

Superior
orbital fissure

Great wing of
sphenoid

Petrous ridge

Clivus   Internal auditory canal

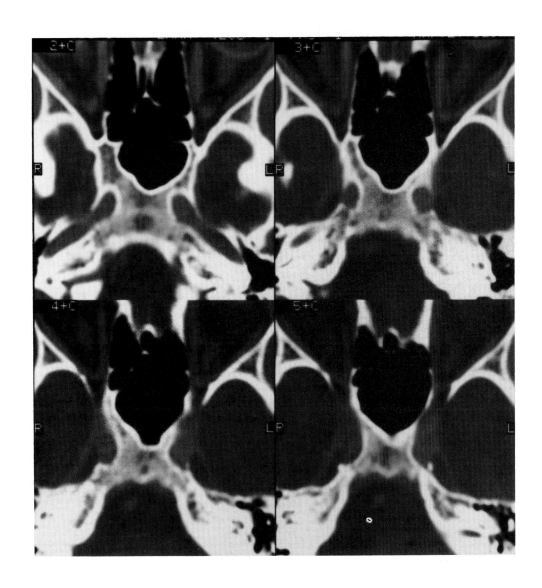

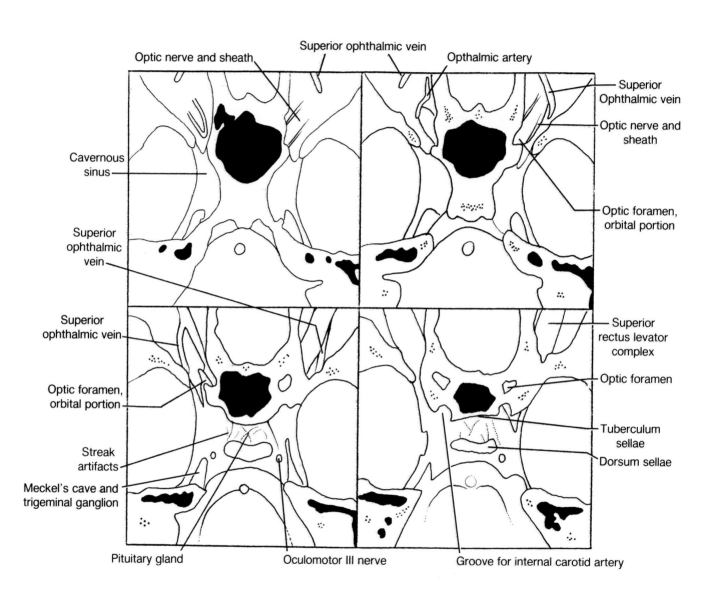

Optic nerve and sheath

Superior ophthalmic vein

Opthalmic artery

Superior Ophthalmic vein

Optic nerve and sheath

Optic foramen, orbital portion

Cavernous sinus

Superior ophthalmic vein

Superior ophthalmic vein

Optic foramen, orbital portion

Superior rectus levator complex

Optic foramen

Tuberculum sellae

Dorsum sellae

Streak artifacts

Meckel's cave and trigeminal ganglion

Pituitary gland

Oculomotor III nerve

Groove for internal carotid artery

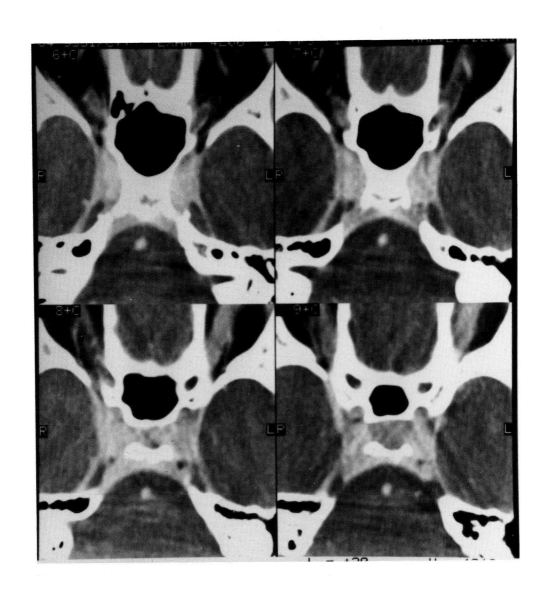

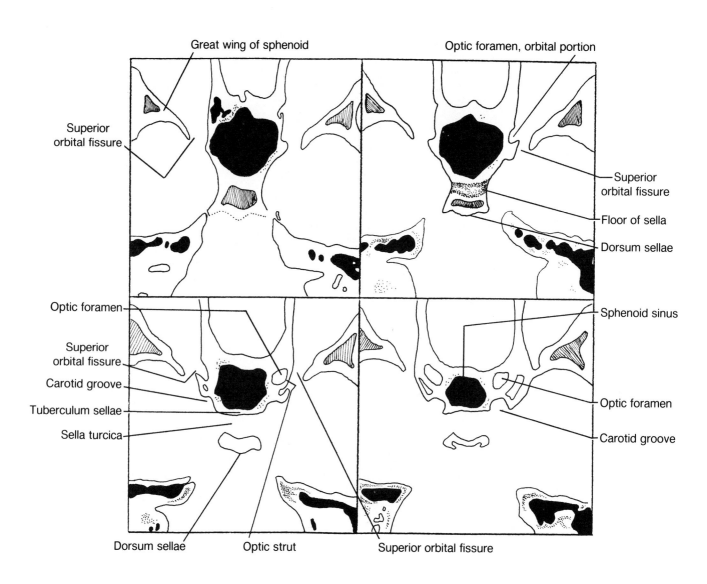

Great wing of sphenoid

Optic foramen, orbital portion

Superior
orbital fissure

Superior
orbital fissure

Floor of sella

Dorsum sellae

Optic foramen

Sphenoid sinus

Superior
orbital fissure

Carotid groove

Tuberculum sellae

Optic foramen

Sella turcica

Carotid groove

Dorsum sellae

Optic strut

Superior orbital fissure

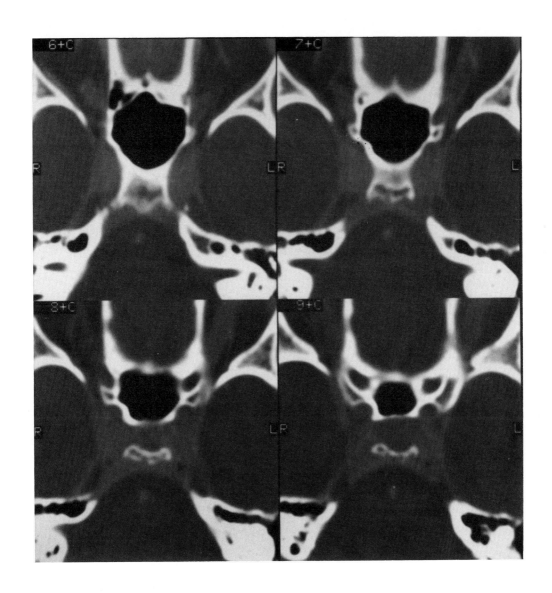

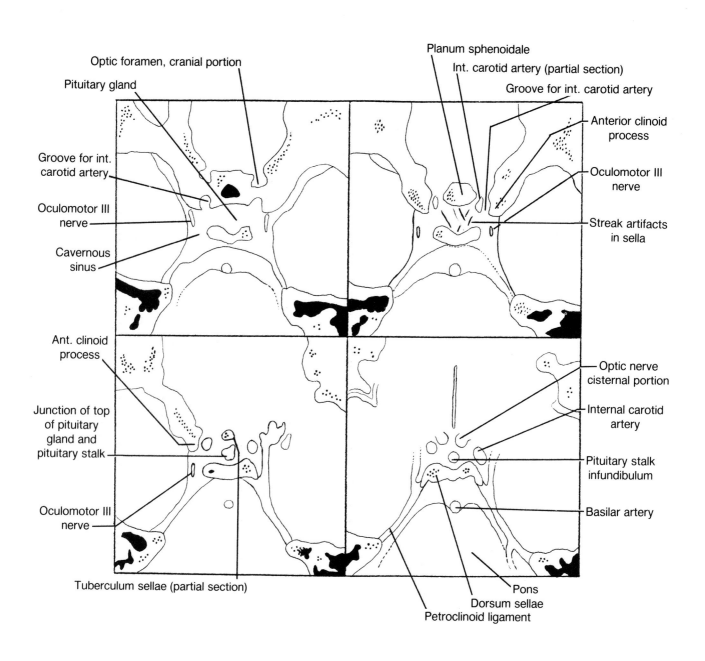

Optic foramen, cranial portion

Pituitary gland

Groove for int.
carotid artery

Oculomotor III
nerve

Cavernous
sinus

Planum sphenoidale

Int. carotid artery (partial section)

Groove for int. carotid artery

Anterior clinoid
process

Oculomotor III
nerve

Streak artifacts
in sella

Ant. clinoid
process

Junction of top
of pituitary
gland and
pituitary stalk

Oculomotor III
nerve

Optic nerve
cisternal portion

Internal carotid
artery

Pituitary stalk
infundibulum

Basilar artery

Tuberculum sellae (partial section)

Pons

Dorsum sellae

Petroclinoid ligament

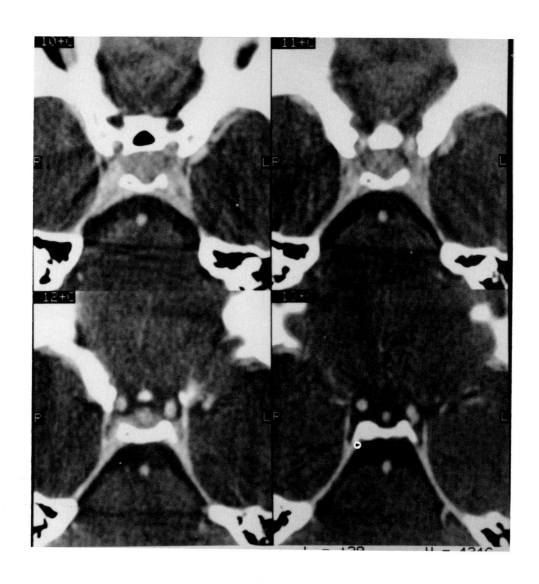

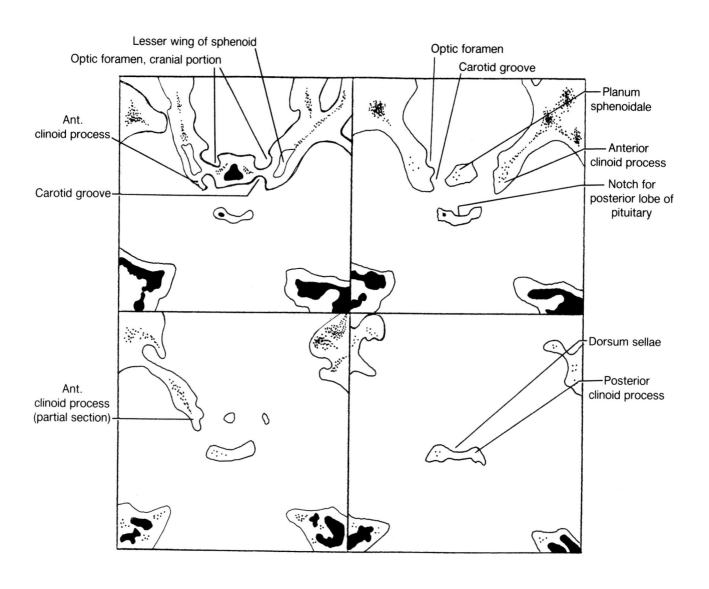

Lesser wing of sphenoid

Optic foramen, cranial portion

Optic foramen

Carotid groove

Ant. clinoid process

Planum sphenoidale

Anterior clinoid process

Carotid groove

Notch for posterior lobe of pituitary

Ant. clinoid process (partial section)

Dorsum sellae

Posterior clinoid process

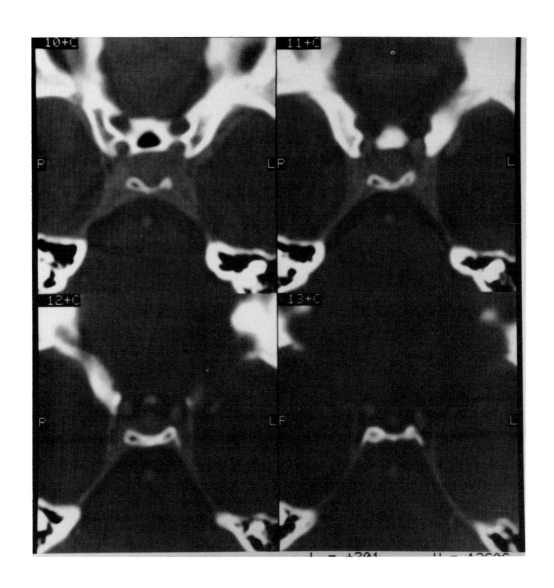

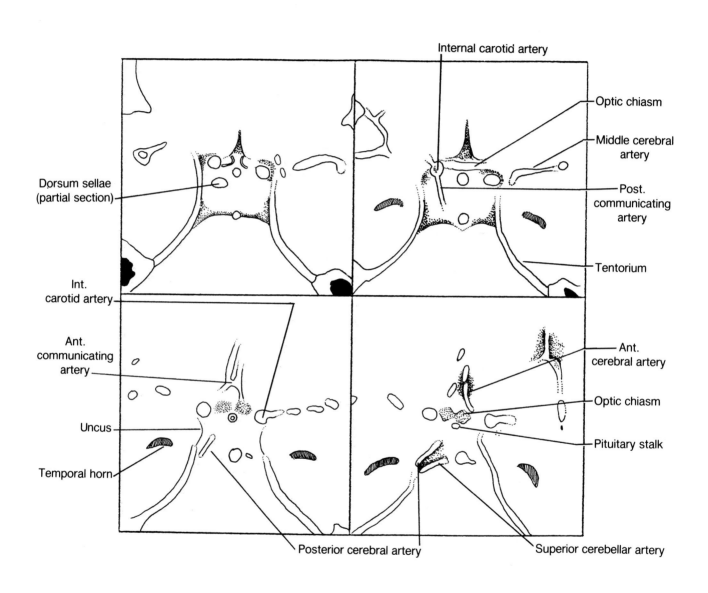

Internal carotid artery

Optic chiasm

Middle cerebral artery

Dorsum sellae (partial section)

Post. communicating artery

Int. carotid artery

Tentorium

Ant. communicating artery

Ant. cerebral artery

Optic chiasm

Pituitary stalk

Uncus

Temporal horn

Posterior cerebral artery

Superior cerebellar artery

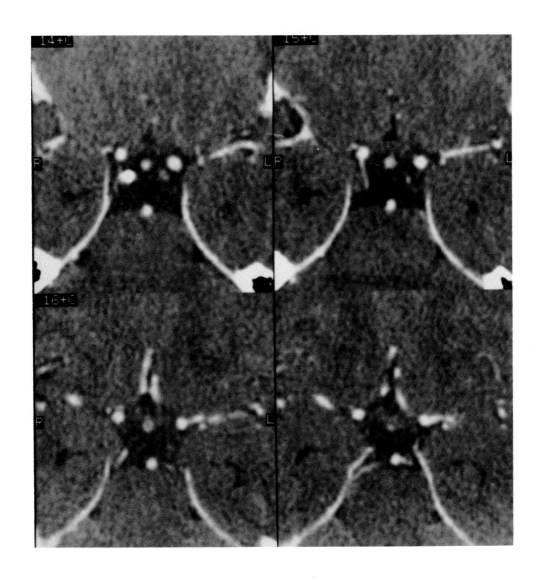

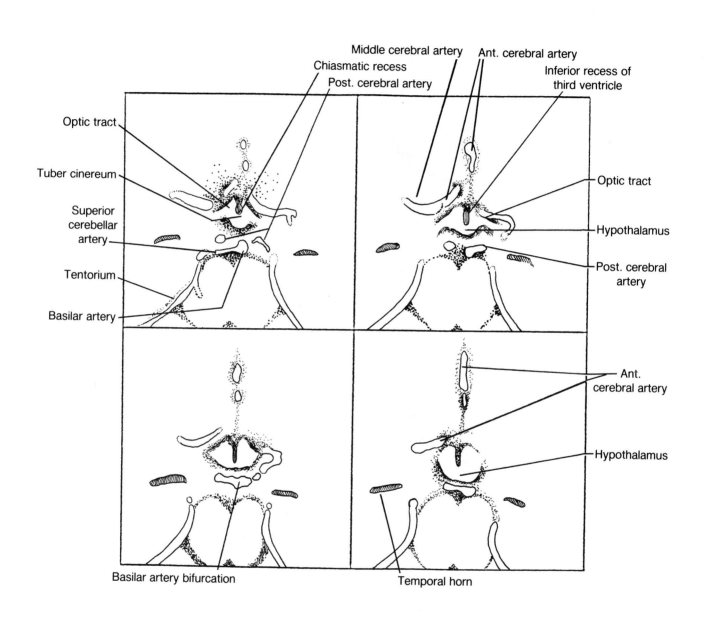

Middle cerebral artery

Chiasmatic recess

Post. cerebral artery

Ant. cerebral artery

Inferior recess of
third ventricle

Optic tract

Tuber cinereum

Superior
cerebellar
artery

Tentorium

Basilar artery

Optic tract

Hypothalamus

Post. cerebral
artery

Ant.
cerebral artery

Hypothalamus

Basilar artery bifurcation

Temporal horn

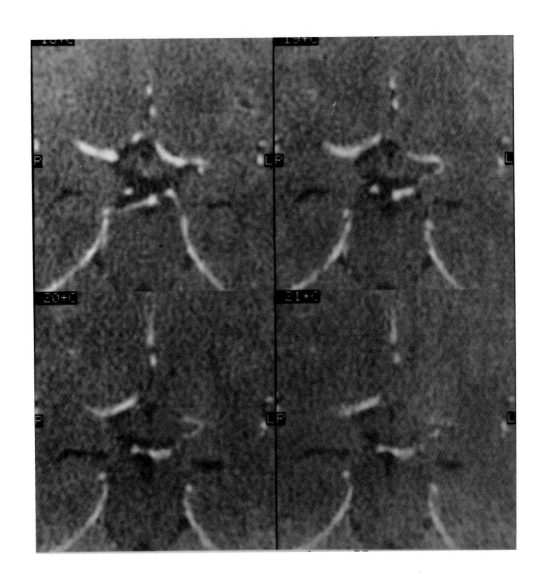

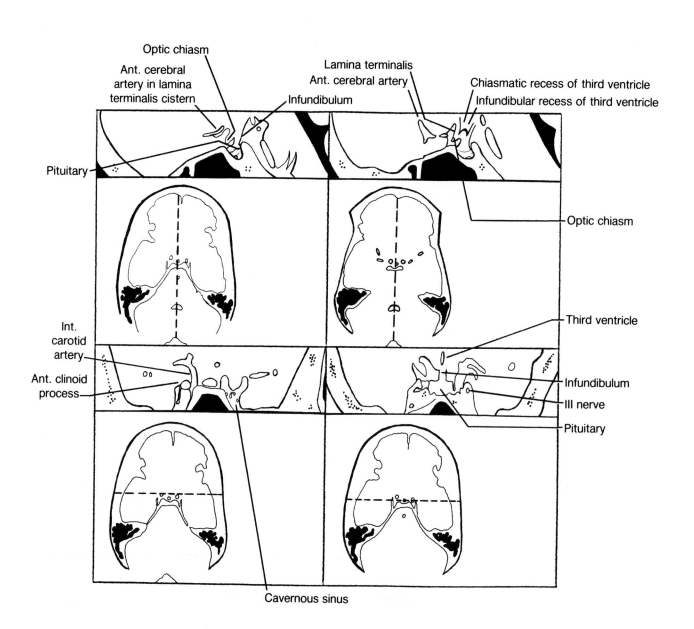

Optic chiasm

Ant. cerebral
artery in lamina
terminalis cistern

Infundibulum

Lamina terminalis
Ant. cerebral artery

Chiasmatic recess of third ventricle
Infundibular recess of third ventricle

Pituitary

Optic chiasm

Int.
carotid
artery

Ant. clinoid
process

Third ventricle

Infundibulum

III nerve

Pituitary

Cavernous sinus

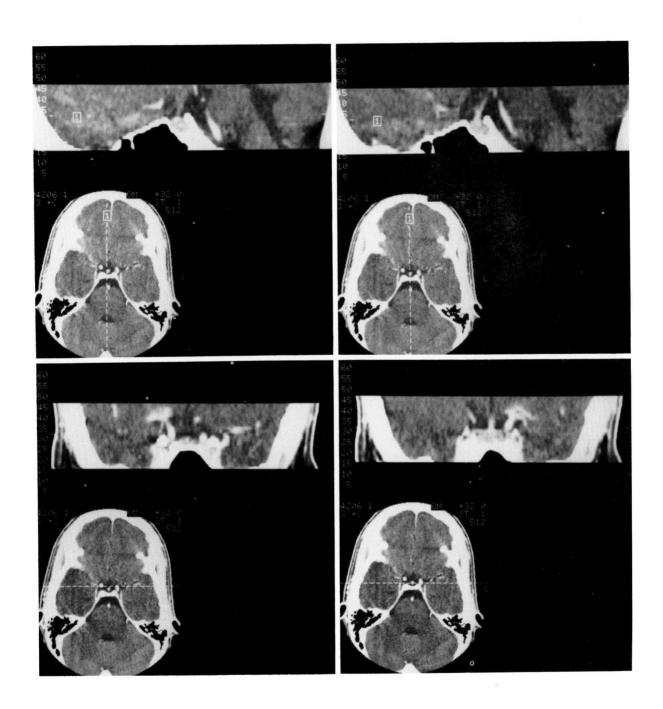

Sella and Juxtasella with Intravenous Contrast: Coronal Plane

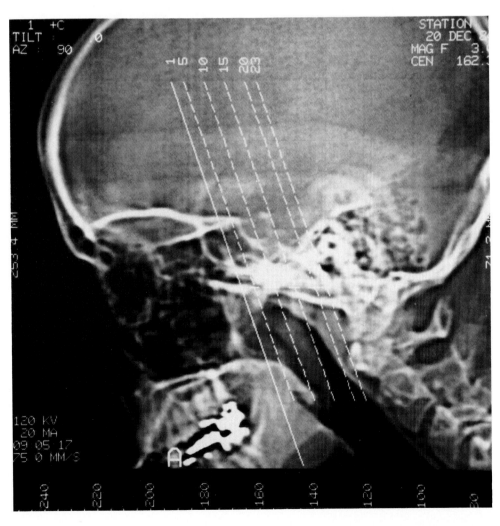

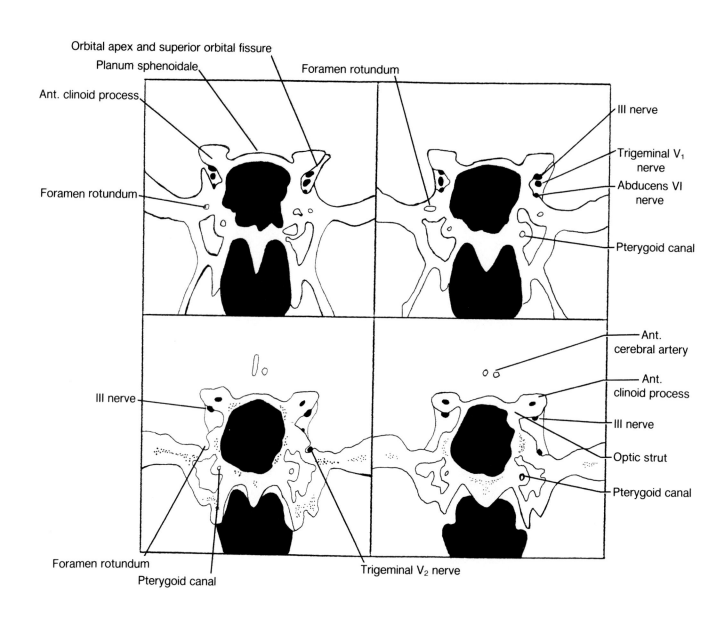

Orbital apex and superior orbital fissure

Planum sphenoidale

Foramen rotundum

Ant. clinoid process

III nerve

Foramen rotundum

Trigeminal V₁ nerve

Abducens VI nerve

Pterygoid canal

Ant. cerebral artery

Ant. clinoid process

III nerve

III nerve

Optic strut

Pterygoid canal

Foramen rotundum

Pterygoid canal

Trigeminal V₂ nerve

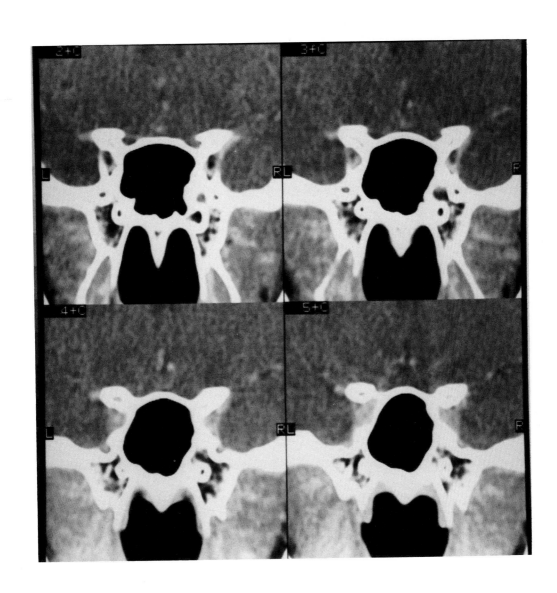

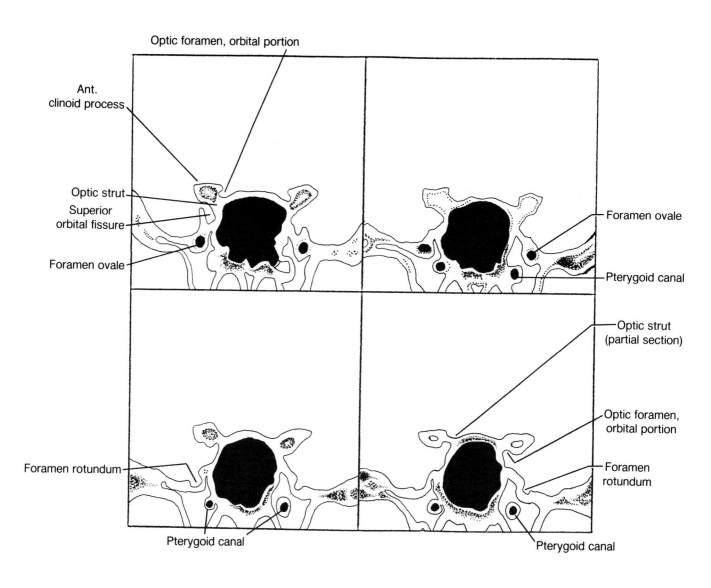

Optic foramen, orbital portion

Ant.
clinoid process

Optic strut
Superior
orbital fissure

Foramen ovale

Foramen ovale

Pterygoid canal

Optic strut
(partial section)

Optic foramen,
orbital portion

Foramen
rotundum

Foramen rotundum

Pterygoid canal

Pterygoid canal

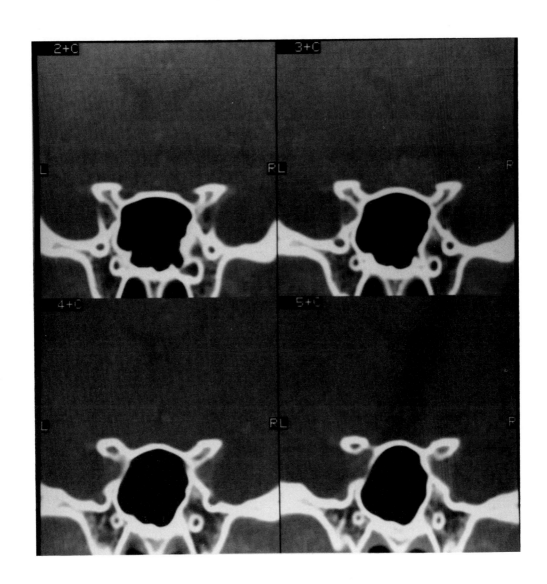

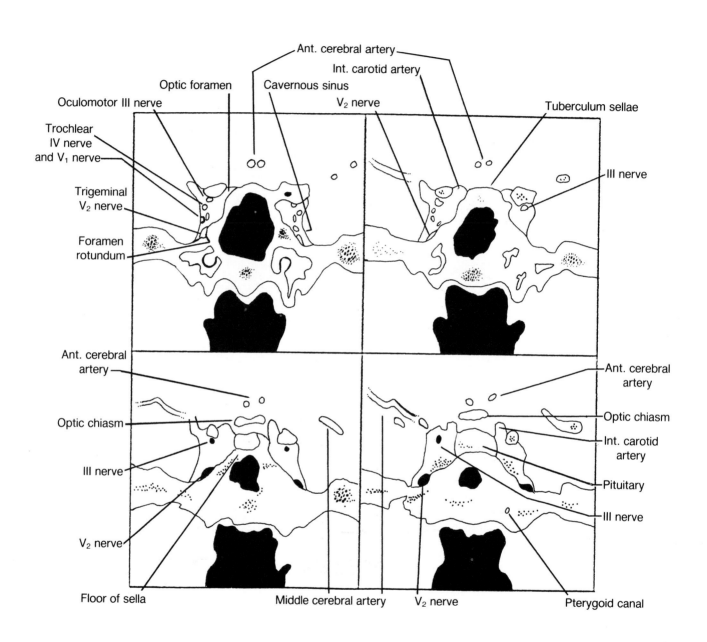

Ant. cerebral artery

Int. carotid artery

Optic foramen

Cavernous sinus

V_2 nerve

Tuberculum sellae

Oculomotor III nerve

Trochlear
IV nerve
and V_1 nerve

III nerve

Trigeminal
V_2 nerve

Foramen
rotundum

Ant. cerebral
artery

Ant. cerebral
artery

Optic chiasm

Optic chiasm

Int. carotid
artery

III nerve

Pituitary

III nerve

V_2 nerve

Floor of sella

Middle cerebral artery

V_2 nerve

Pterygoid canal

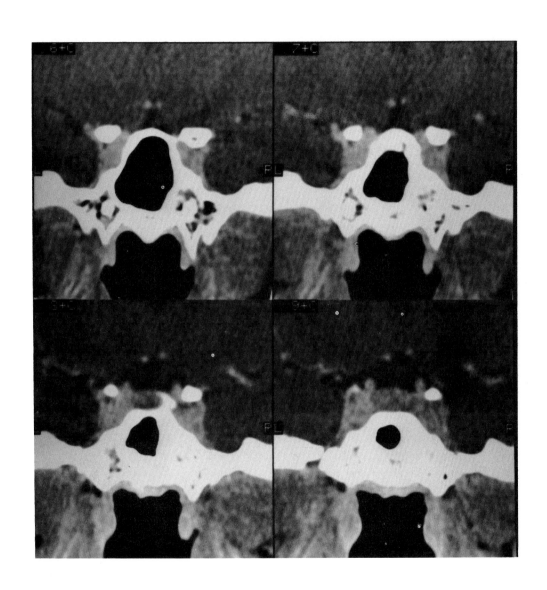

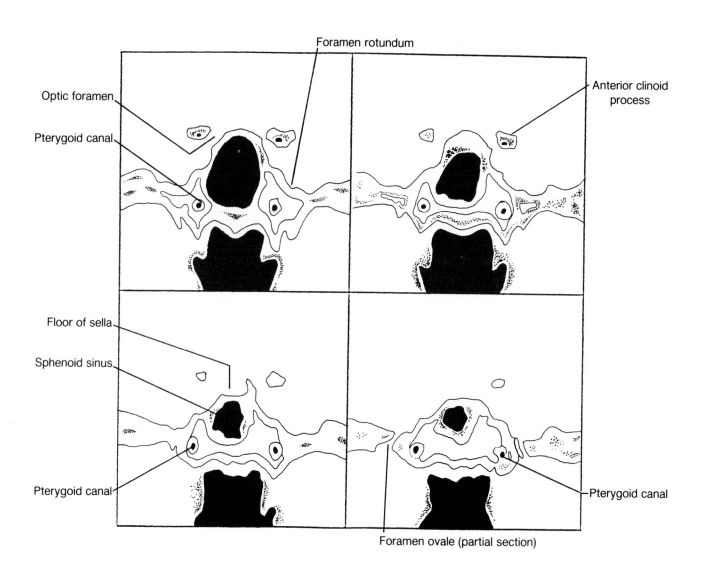

Foramen rotundum

Optic foramen

Pterygoid canal

Anterior clinoid process

Floor of sella

Sphenoid sinus

Pterygoid canal

Pterygoid canal

Foramen ovale (partial section)

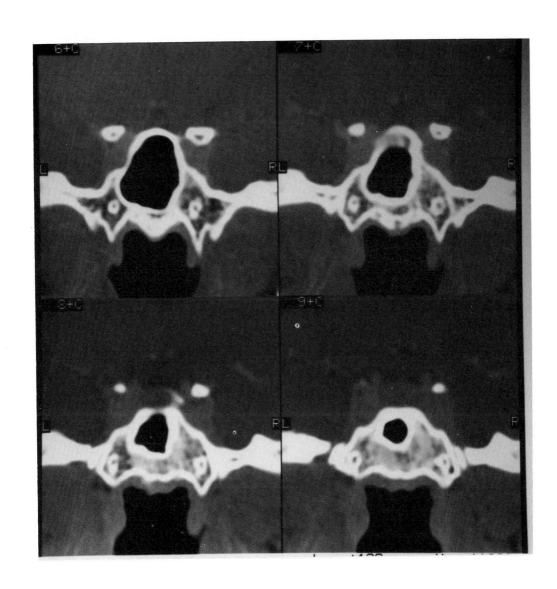

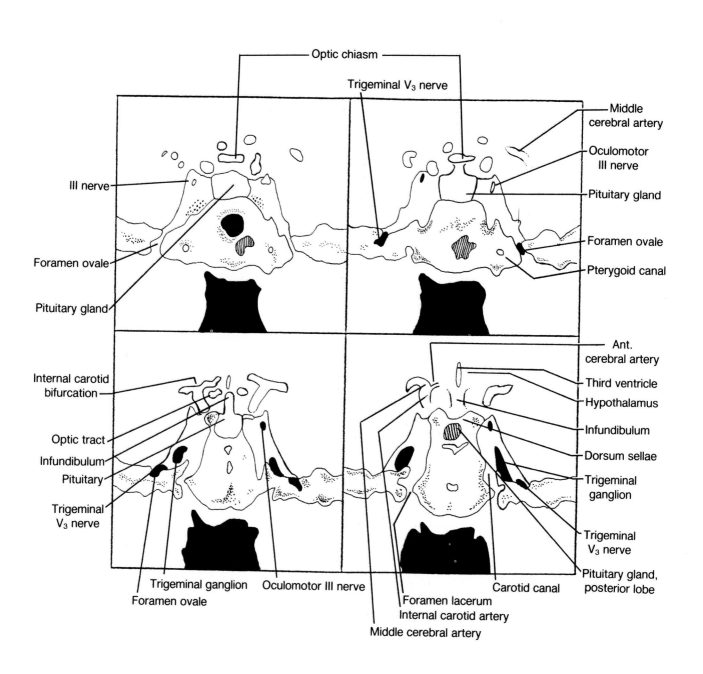

Optic chiasm

Trigeminal V₃ nerve

Middle cerebral artery

Oculomotor III nerve

III nerve

Pituitary gland

Foramen ovale

Foramen ovale

Pterygoid canal

Pituitary gland

Internal carotid bifurcation

Ant. cerebral artery

Third ventricle

Hypothalamus

Optic tract

Infundibulum

Infundibulum

Pituitary

Dorsum sellae

Trigeminal V₃ nerve

Trigeminal ganglion

Trigeminal V₃ nerve

Trigeminal ganglion

Oculomotor III nerve

Carotid canal

Pituitary gland, posterior lobe

Foramen ovale

Foramen lacerum

Internal carotid artery

Middle cerebral artery

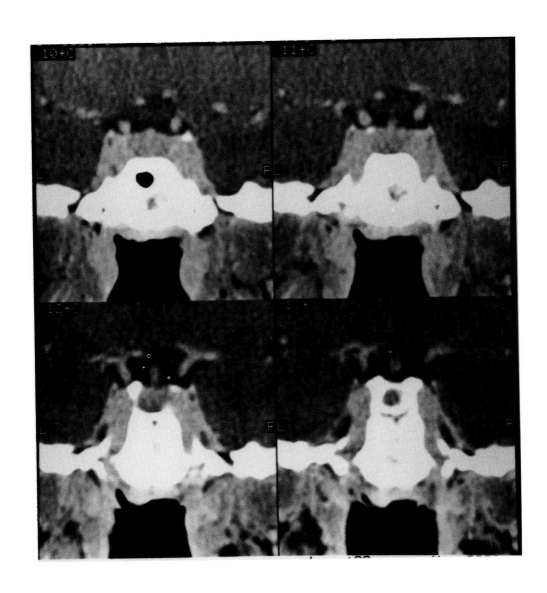

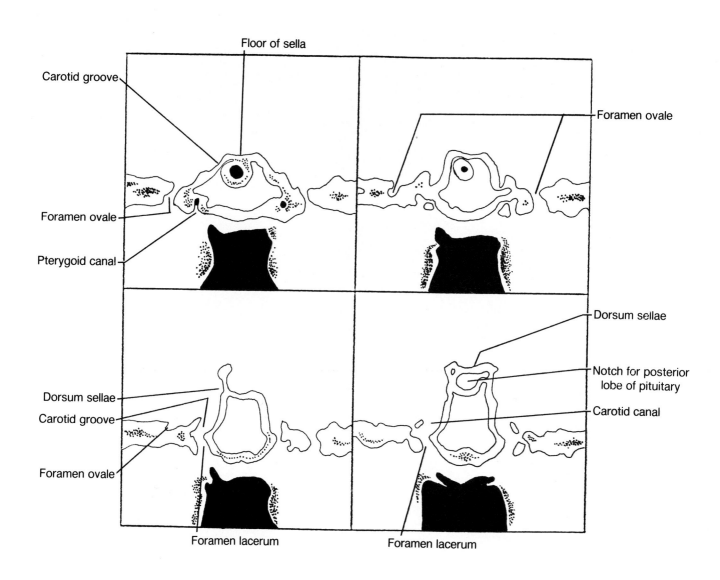

Floor of sella

Carotid groove

Foramen ovale

Foramen ovale

Pterygoid canal

Dorsum sellae

Notch for posterior lobe of pituitary

Carotid canal

Dorsum sellae

Carotid groove

Foramen ovale

Foramen lacerum

Foramen lacerum

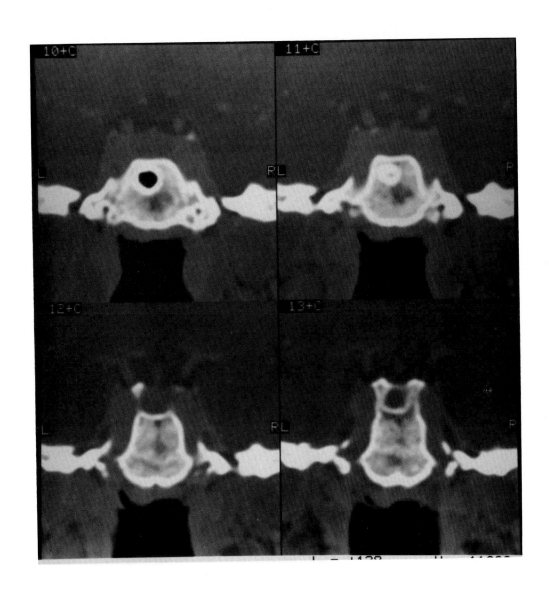

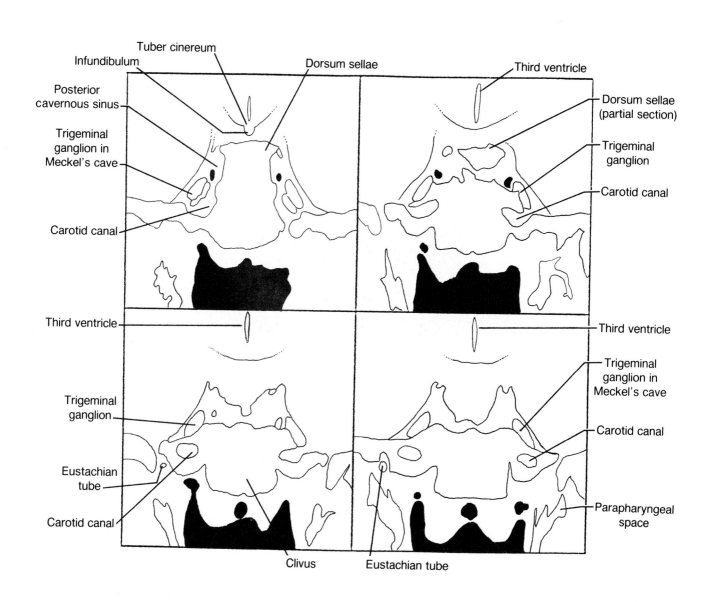

Tuber cinereum

Infundibulum

Dorsum sellae

Third ventricle

Posterior cavernous sinus

Dorsum sellae (partial section)

Trigeminal ganglion in Meckel's cave

Trigeminal ganglion

Carotid canal

Carotid canal

Third ventricle

Third ventricle

Trigeminal ganglion

Trigeminal ganglion in Meckel's cave

Eustachian tube

Carotid canal

Carotid canal

Parapharyngeal space

Clivus

Eustachian tube

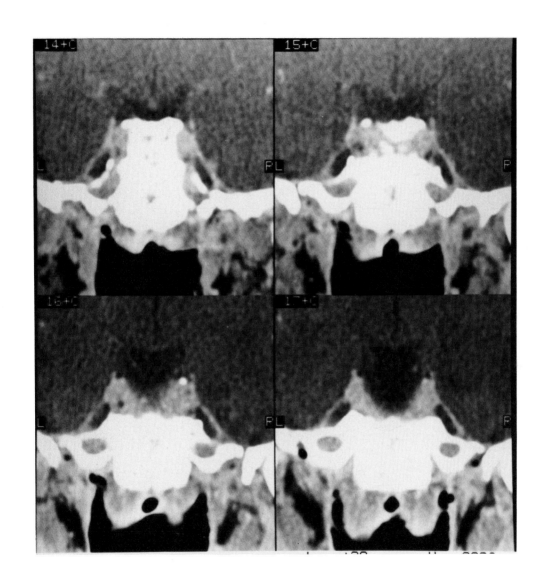

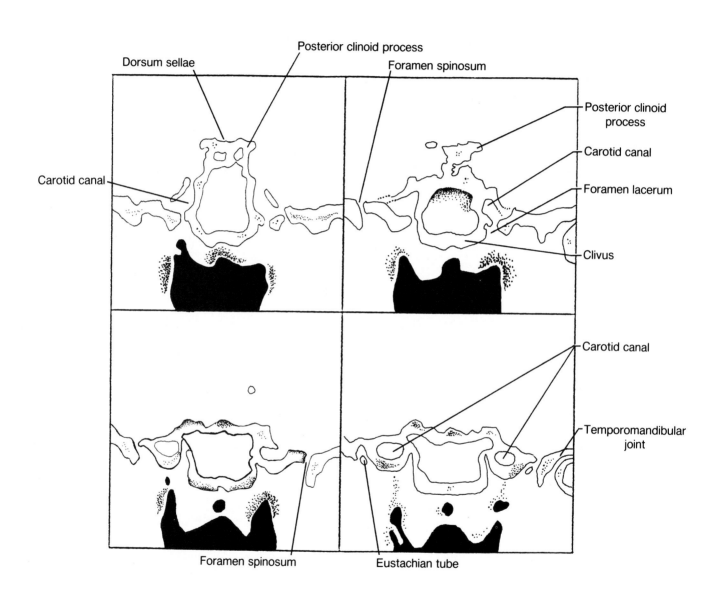

Dorsum sellae

Posterior clinoid process

Foramen spinosum

Posterior clinoid process

Carotid canal

Carotid canal

Foramen lacerum

Clivus

Carotid canal

Temporomandibular joint

Foramen spinosum

Eustachian tube

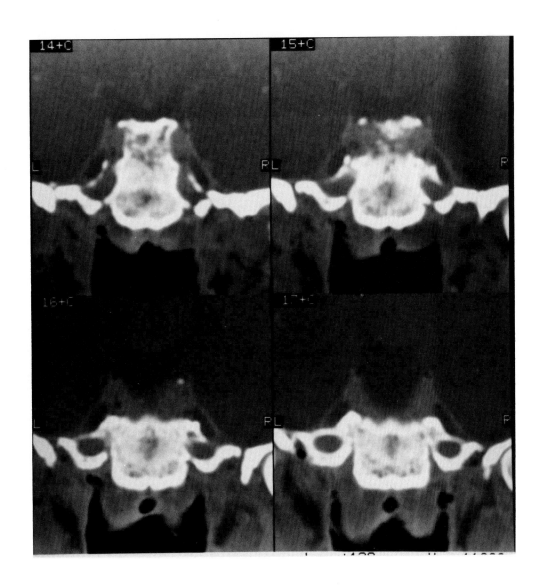

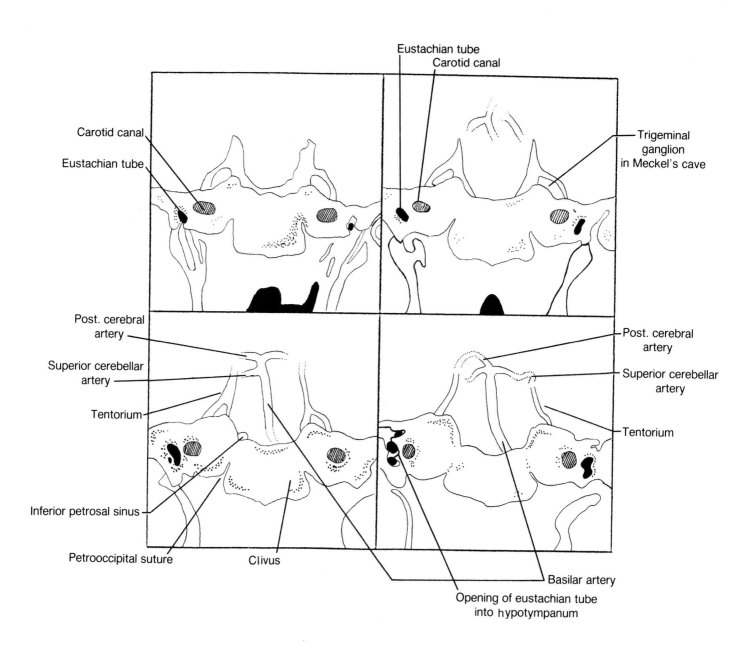

Eustachian tube
Carotid canal

Carotid canal
Eustachian tube

Trigeminal ganglion in Meckel's cave

Post. cerebral artery

Superior cerebellar artery

Tentorium

Inferior petrosal sinus

Petrooccipital suture

Clivus

Post. cerebral artery

Superior cerebellar artery

Tentorium

Basilar artery

Opening of eustachian tube into hypotympanum

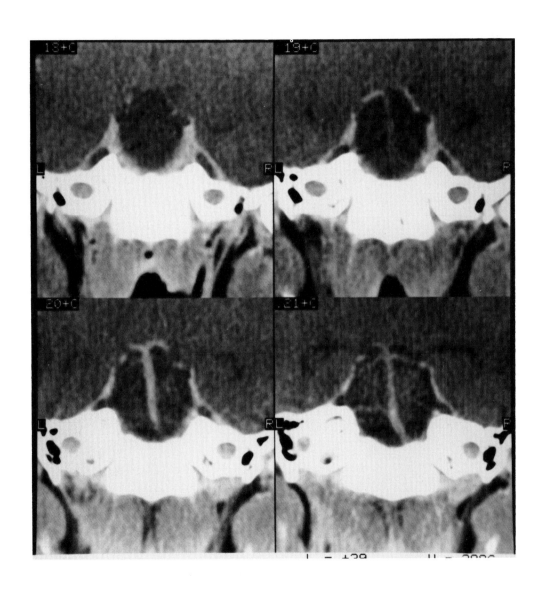

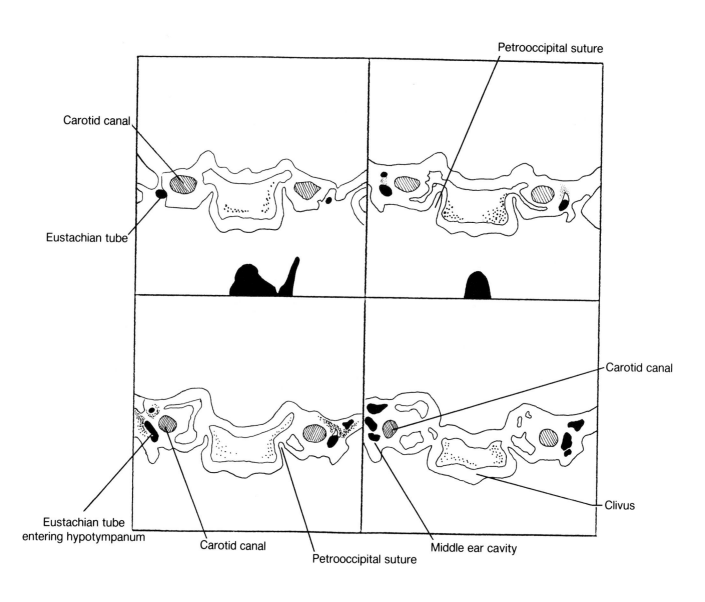

Petrooccipital suture

Carotid canal

Eustachian tube

Eustachian tube
entering hypotympanum

Carotid canal

Petrooccipital suture

Middle ear cavity

Carotid canal

Clivus

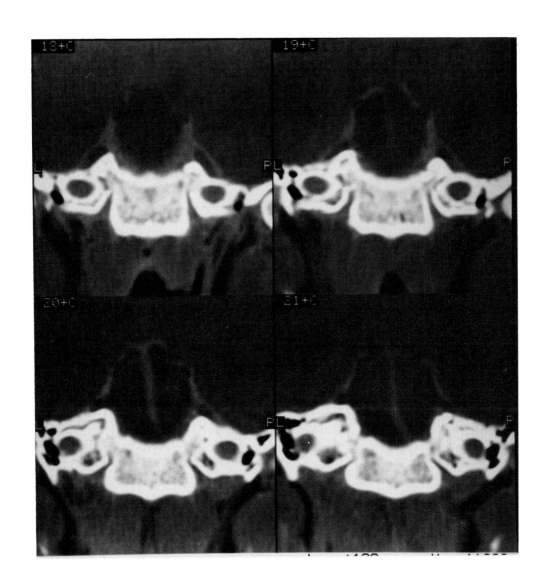

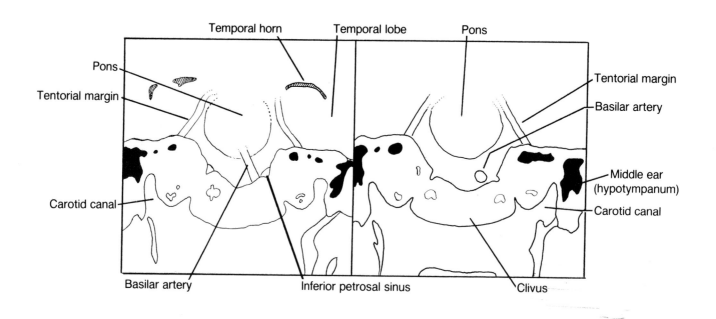

Temporal horn

Temporal lobe

Pons

Pons

Tentorial margin

Tentorial margin

Basilar artery

Middle ear
(hypotympanum)

Carotid canal

Carotid canal

Basilar artery

Inferior petrosal sinus

Clivus

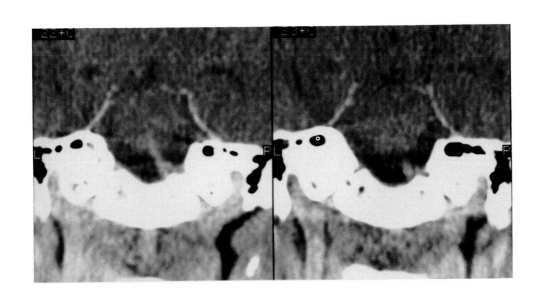

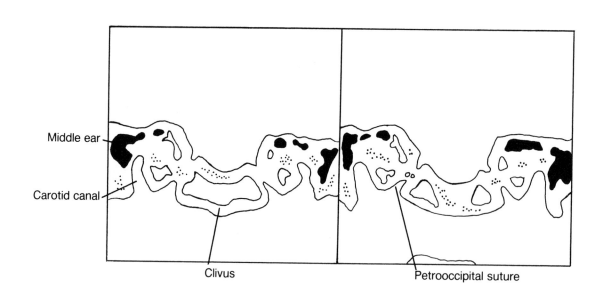

Middle ear

Carotid canal

Clivus

Petrooccipital suture

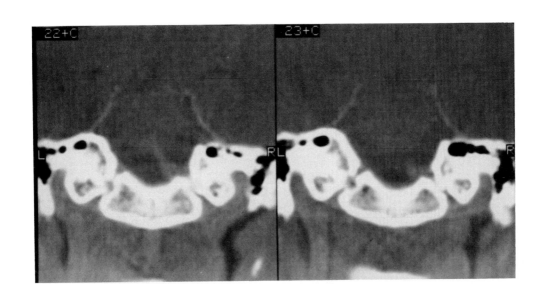

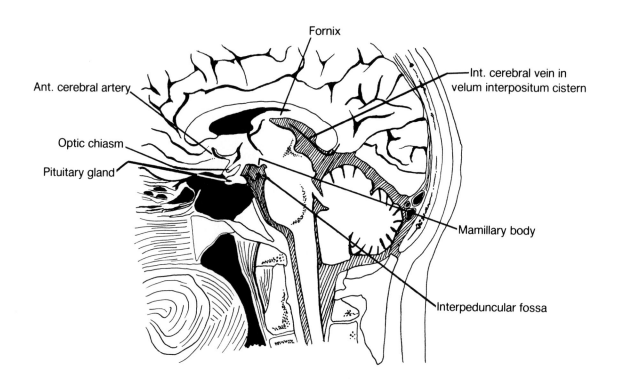

Fornix

Int. cerebral vein in
velum interpositum cistern

Ant. cerebral artery

Optic chiasm

Pituitary gland

Mamillary body

Interpeduncular fossa

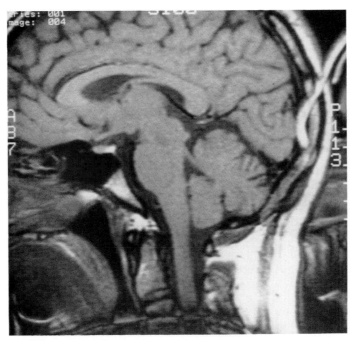

Midsagittal MRI of the brain demonstrating the sellar and juxtasellar area.

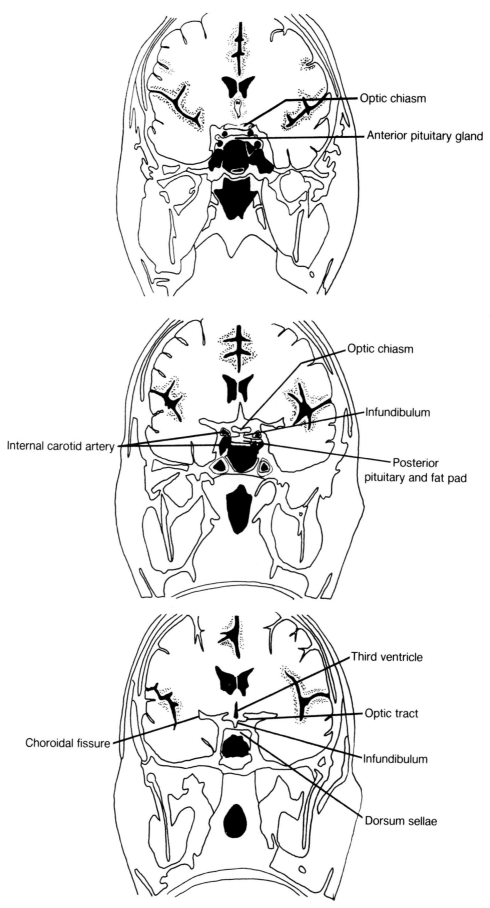

Optic chiasm

Anterior pituitary gland

Optic chiasm

Infundibulum

Internal carotid artery

Posterior
pituitary and fat pad

Third ventricle

Optic tract

Choroidal fissure

Infundibulum

Dorsum sellae

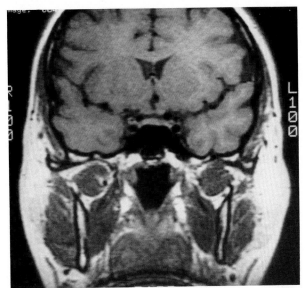

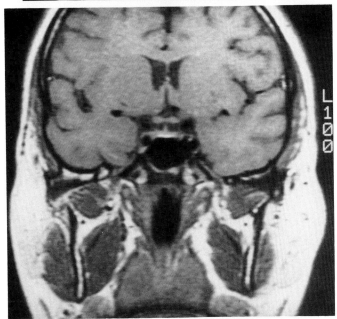

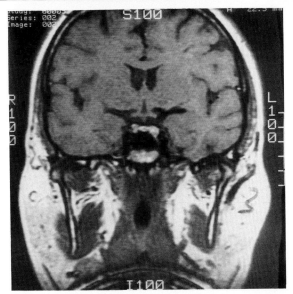

Coronal MRI of the brain at the level of the sella turcica.

3 Orbit

In order to visualize the optic nerve in its entirety and to better visualize the bony optic canal, a scan plane at approximately −30° to Reid's base line has been chosen. If accurately reformatted images are desired, the gantry should not be tilted and the patient's head must be positioned to achieve the desired scan plane. This may not be practical in trauma cases, and is specifically contraindicated in patients with cervical spine injury. If neck injury exists and direct coronal evaluation is not practical, 1.5-mm sections through the orbital floor with 3-mm sections above this will provide more accurate reformatted images through the orbital floor. If the orbit is to be evaluated along with the midface structures, a scan plane more parallel to Reid's base line will be required. Generally, 3-mm thick sections at 3-mm intervals are used. When possible, direct coronal examination is recommended to obtain optimal definition of the orbital floor.

Sections of 1.5 mm through the optic canals may be necessary in trauma cases in order to identify small fragments or occult fractures. Details of the orbital apex and optic canal region with 1.5-mm axial and coronal sections are included in Chapter 2 (Sella and Juxtasella). Coronal anatomy of the orbit is included in Chapter 4 (Paranasal Sinuses and Nasopharynx).

Most orbital scans are performed unenhanced, with intravenous contrast used only for specific indications.

Soft tissue and bone window images are illustrated in this chapter. The sagittal reformatted images are not from the same individual as the axial images, since the gantry tilt used to obtain the axial images would cause distorted reformatted images. The sagittal reformatted images shown here are designed to compare a true sagittal plane with an oblique plane through the optic nerve. The true sagittal plane does not demonstrate the entire length of the optic nerve, whereas the nerve is well shown in the oblique plane.

Orbit with Intravenous Contrast

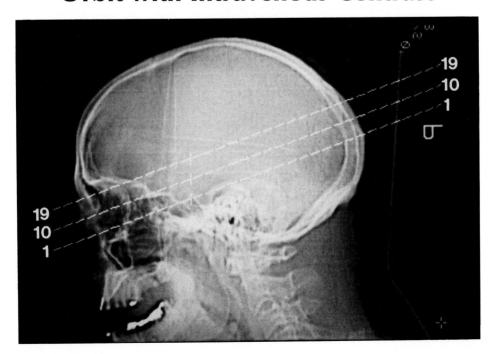

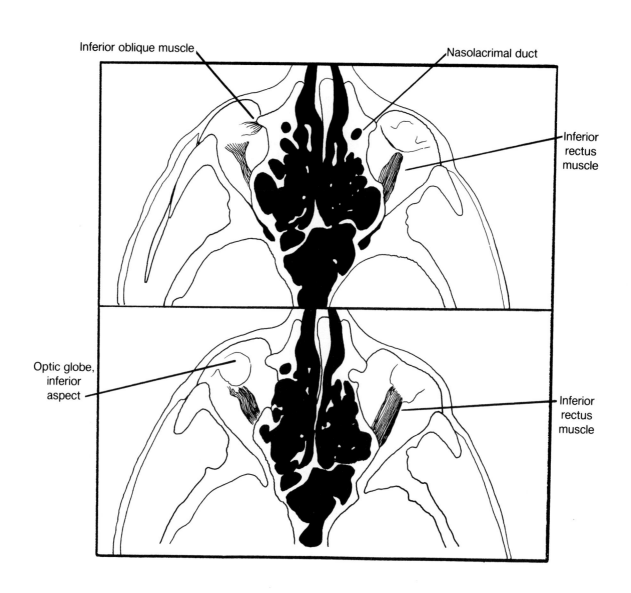

Inferior oblique muscle

Nasolacrimal duct

Inferior rectus muscle

Optic globe, inferior aspect

Inferior rectus muscle

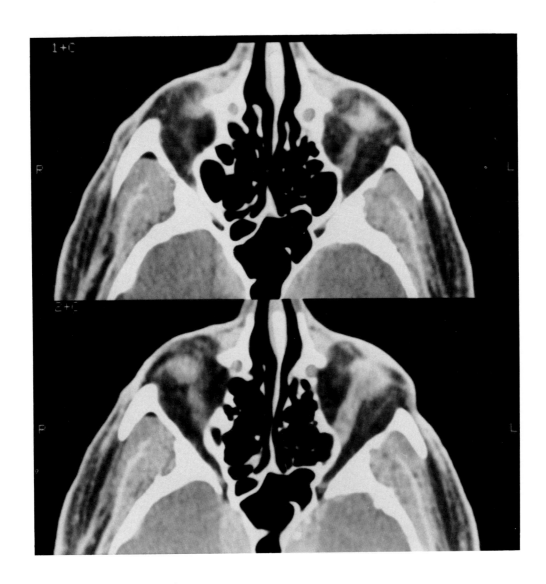

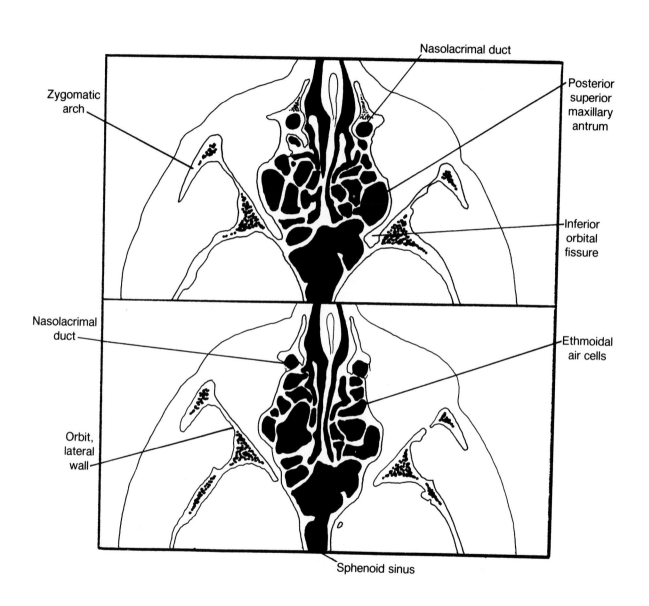

Nasolacrimal duct

Zygomatic
arch

Posterior
superior
maxillary
antrum

Inferior
orbital
fissure

Nasolacrimal
duct

Ethmoidal
air cells

Orbit,
lateral
wall

Sphenoid sinus

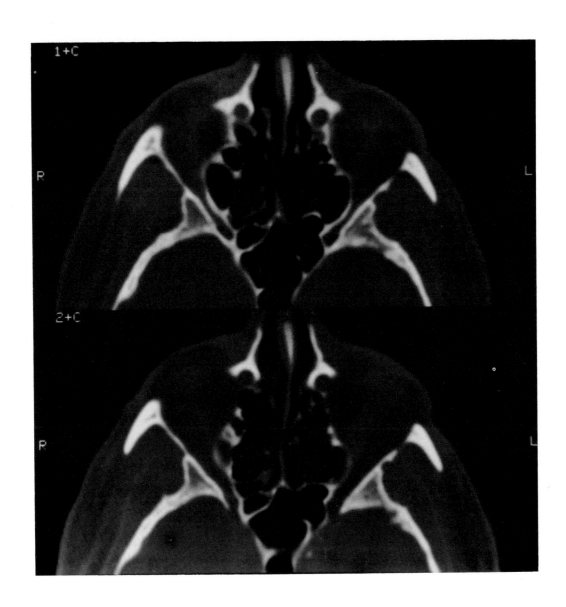

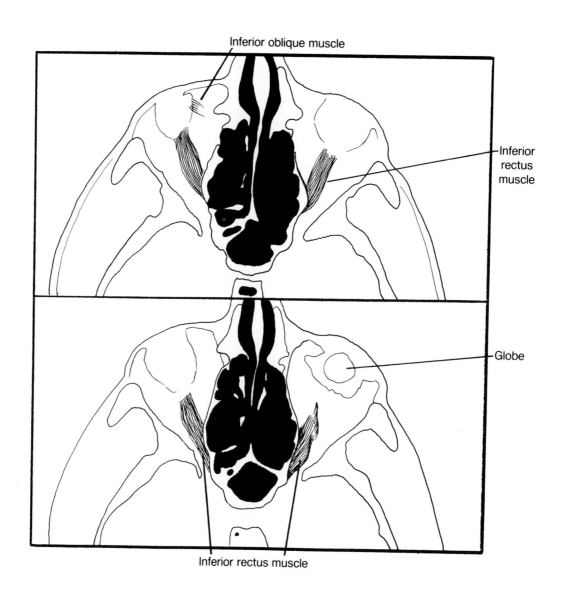

Inferior oblique muscle

Inferior rectus muscle

Globe

Inferior rectus muscle

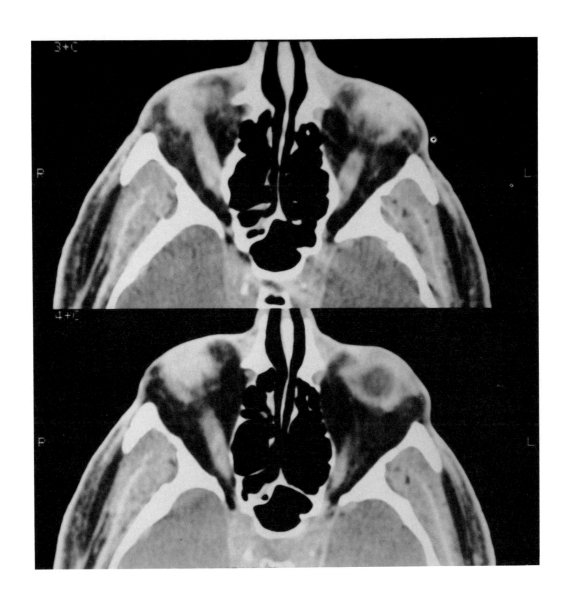

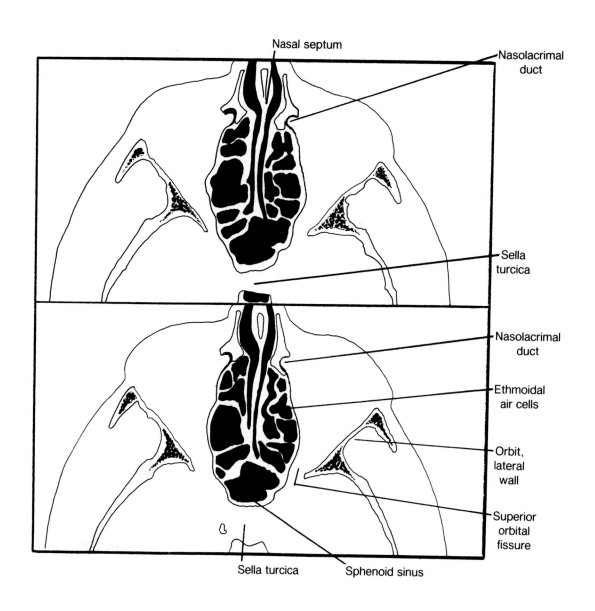

Nasal septum

Nasolacrimal
duct

Sella
turcica

Nasolacrimal
duct

Ethmoidal
air cells

Orbit,
lateral
wall

Superior
orbital
fissure

Sella turcica

Sphenoid sinus

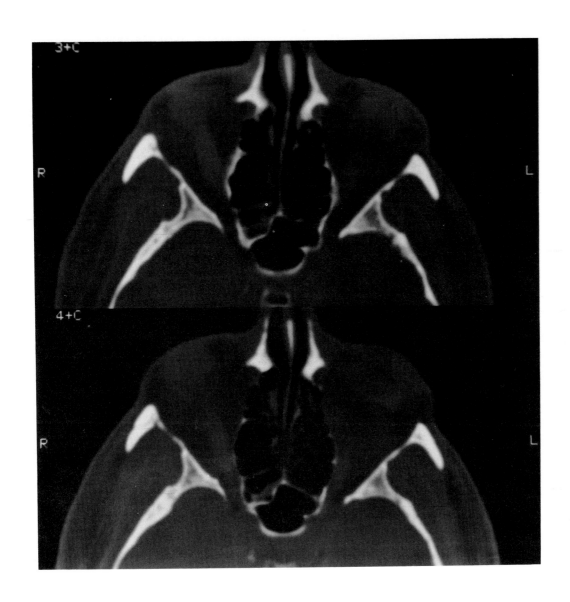

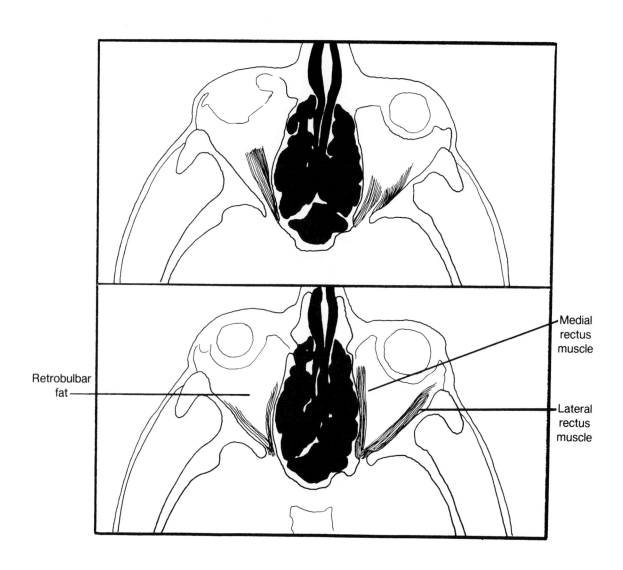

Retrobulbar
fat

Medial
rectus
muscle

Lateral
rectus
muscle

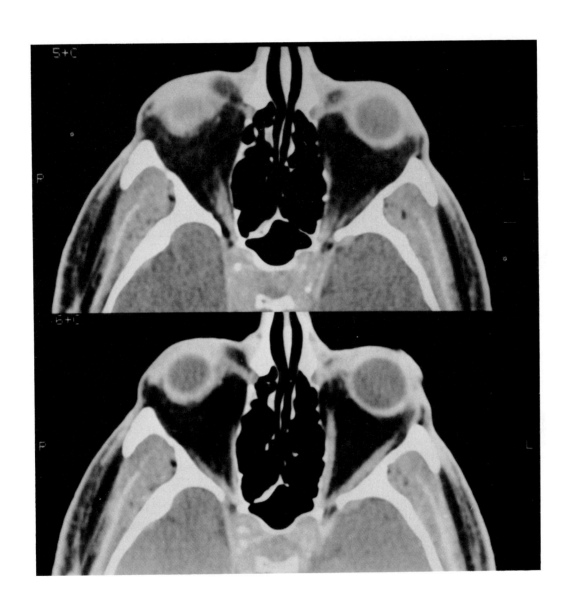

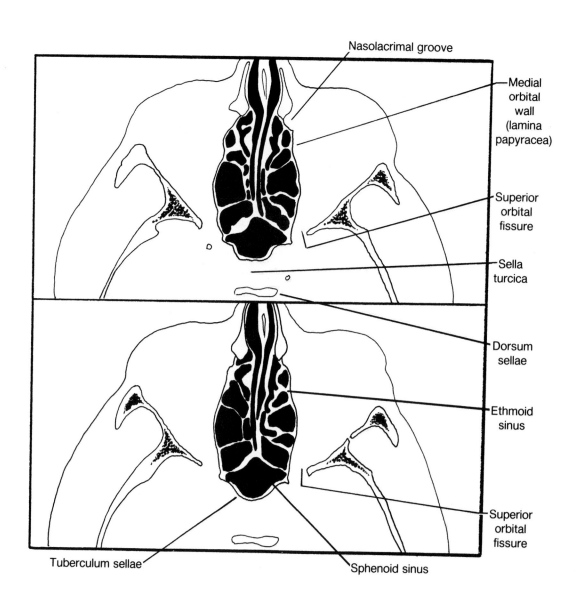

Nasolacrimal groove

Medial
orbital
wall
(lamina
papyracea)

Superior
orbital
fissure

Sella
turcica

Dorsum
sellae

Ethmoid
sinus

Superior
orbital
fissure

Tuberculum sellae

Sphenoid sinus

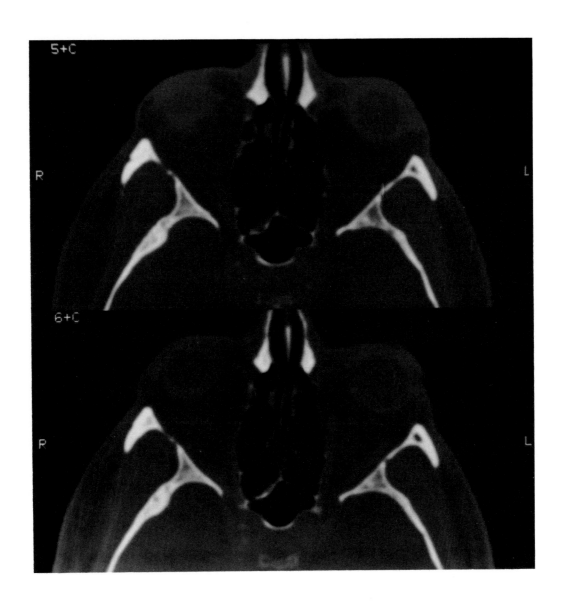

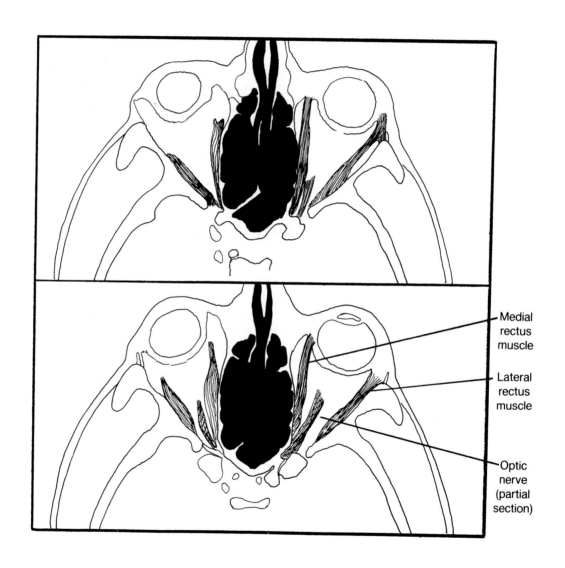

Medial
rectus
muscle

Lateral
rectus
muscle

Optic
nerve
(partial
section)

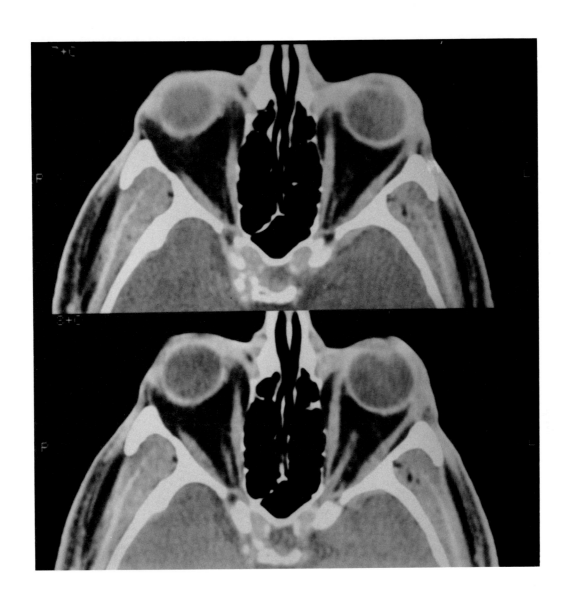

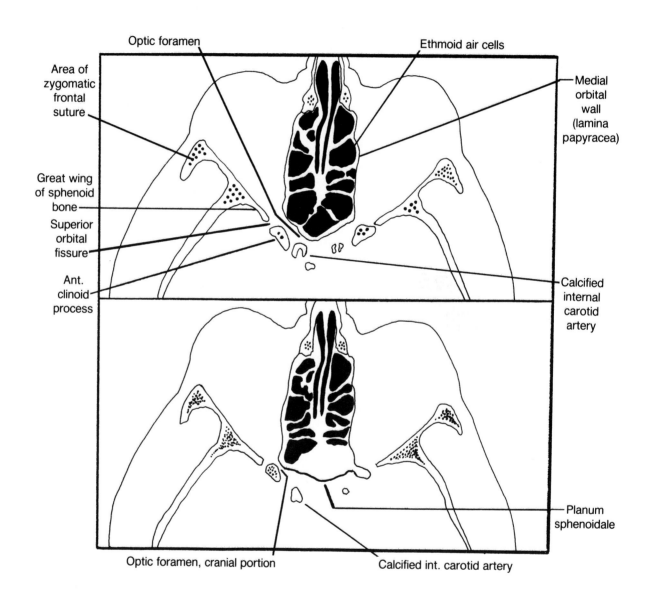

Optic foramen

Ethmoid air cells

Area of zygomatic frontal suture

Medial orbital wall (lamina papyracea)

Great wing of sphenoid bone

Superior orbital fissure

Ant. clinoid process

Calcified internal carotid artery

Optic foramen, cranial portion

Calcified int. carotid artery

Planum sphenoidale

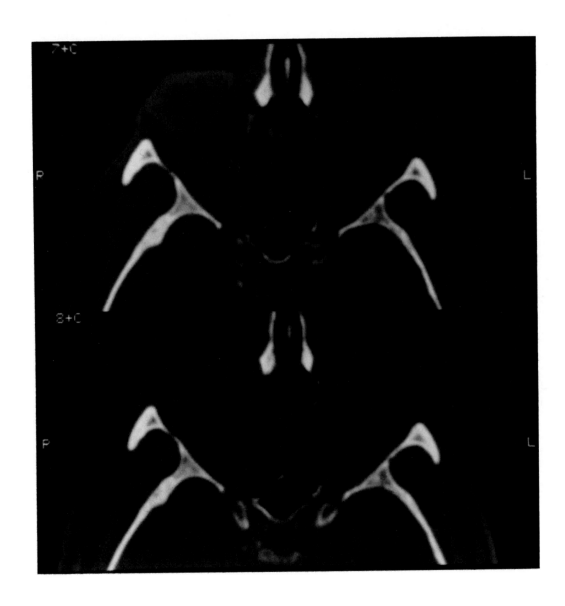

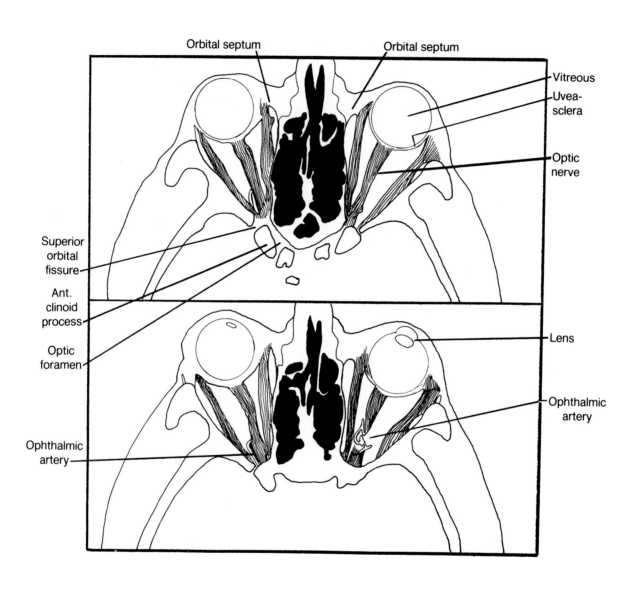

Orbital septum

Orbital septum

Vitreous

Uvea-sclera

Optic nerve

Superior orbital fissure

Ant. clinoid process

Optic foramen

Ophthalmic artery

Lens

Ophthalmic artery

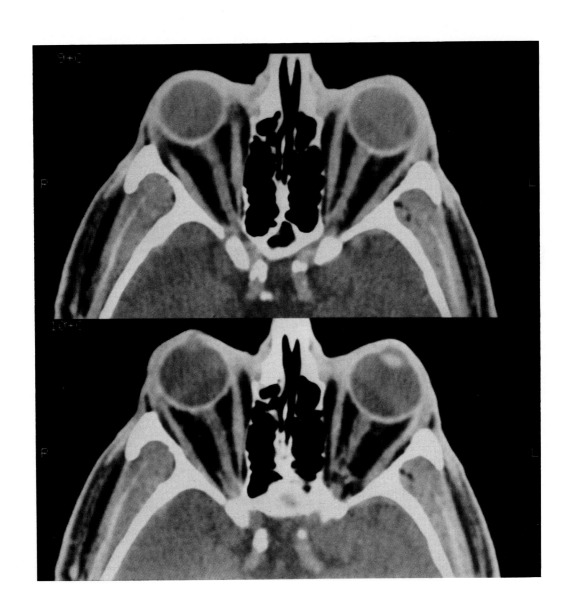

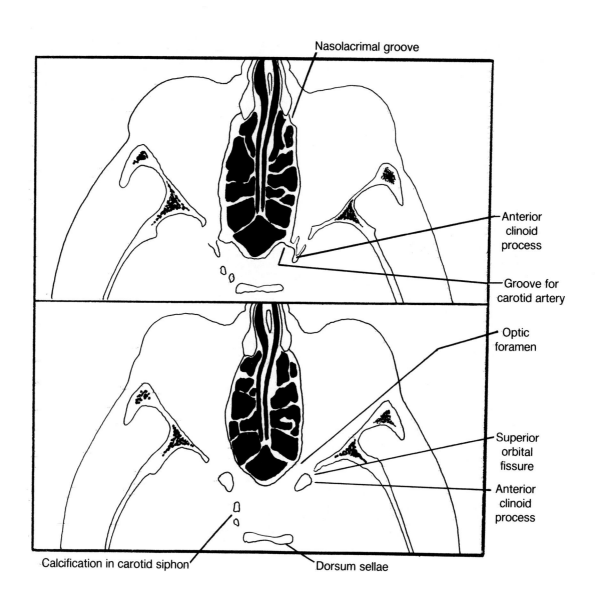

Nasolacrimal groove

Anterior clinoid process

Groove for carotid artery

Optic foramen

Superior orbital fissure

Anterior clinoid process

Calcification in carotid siphon

Dorsum sellae

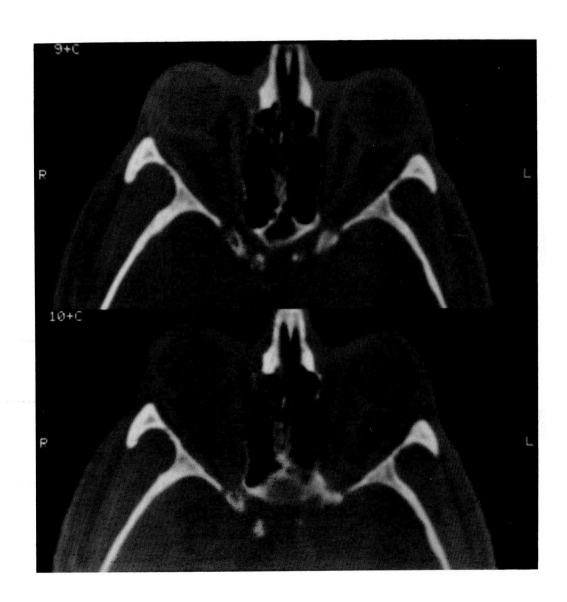

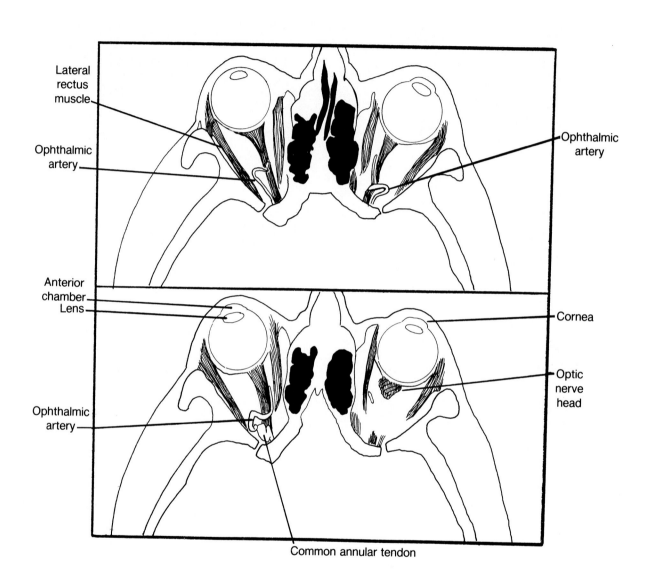

Lateral
rectus
muscle

Ophthalmic
artery

Anterior
chamber
Lens

Ophthalmic
artery

Ophthalmic
artery

Cornea

Optic
nerve
head

Common annular tendon

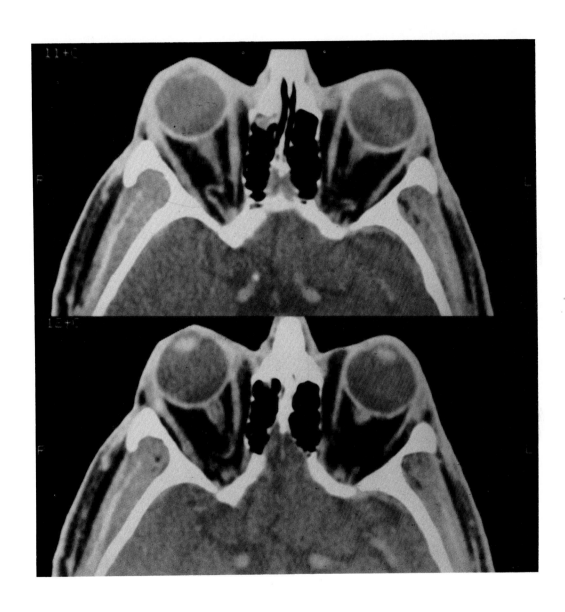

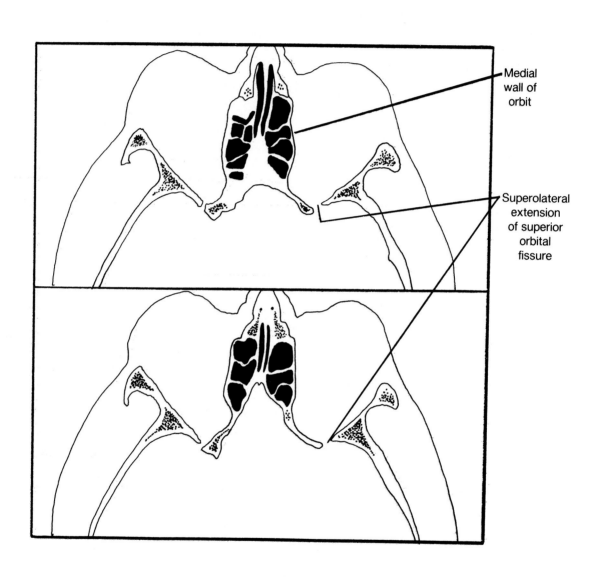

Medial
wall of
orbit

Superolateral
extension
of superior
orbital
fissure

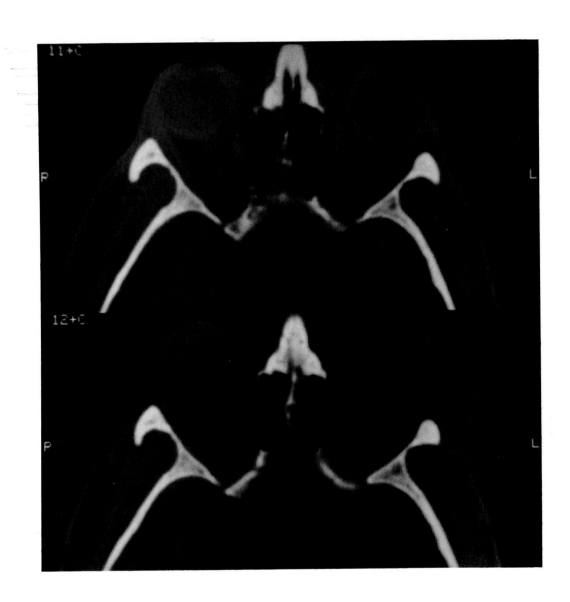

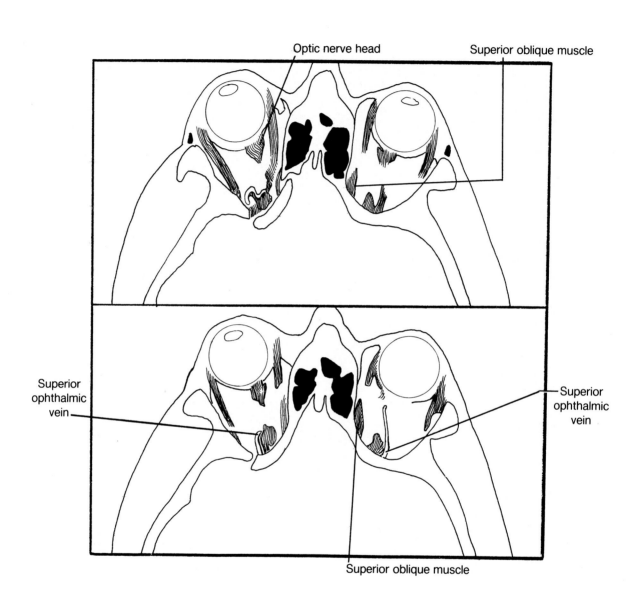

Optic nerve head

Superior oblique muscle

Superior
ophthalmic
vein

Superior
ophthalmic
vein

Superior oblique muscle

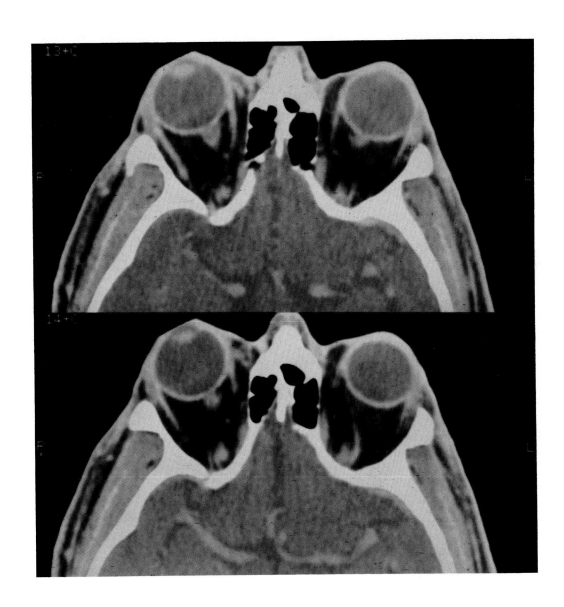

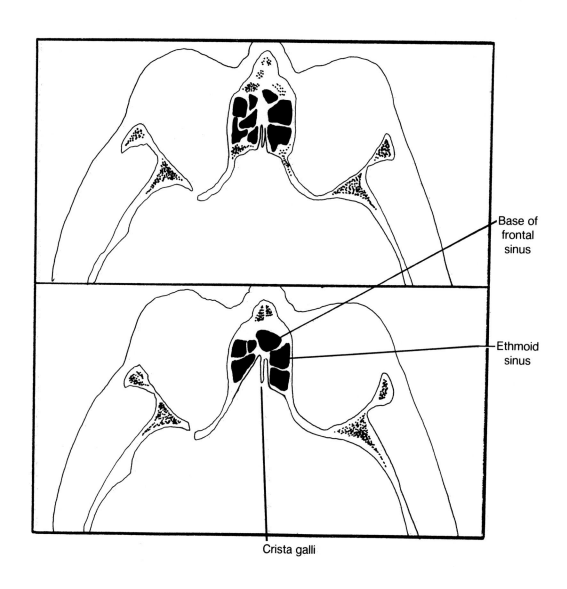

Base of
frontal
sinus

Ethmoid
sinus

Crista galli

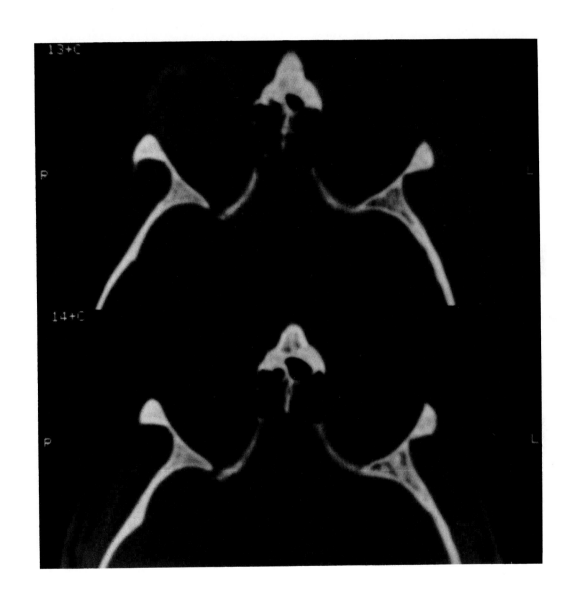

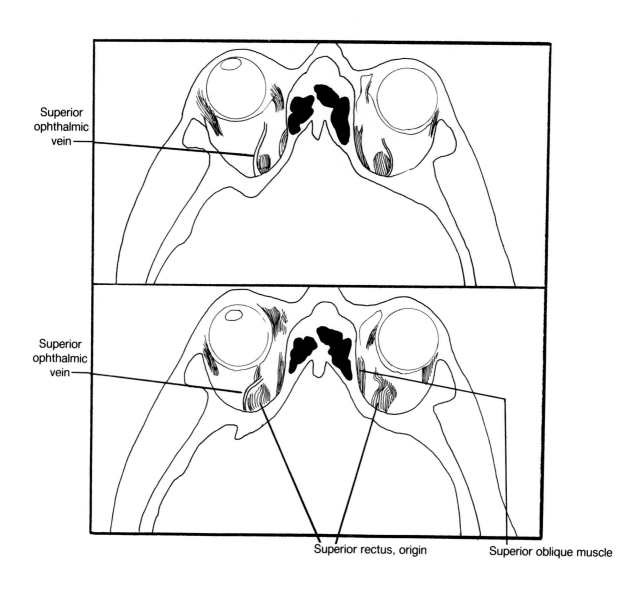

Superior
ophthalmic
vein

Superior
ophthalmic
vein

Superior rectus, origin

Superior oblique muscle

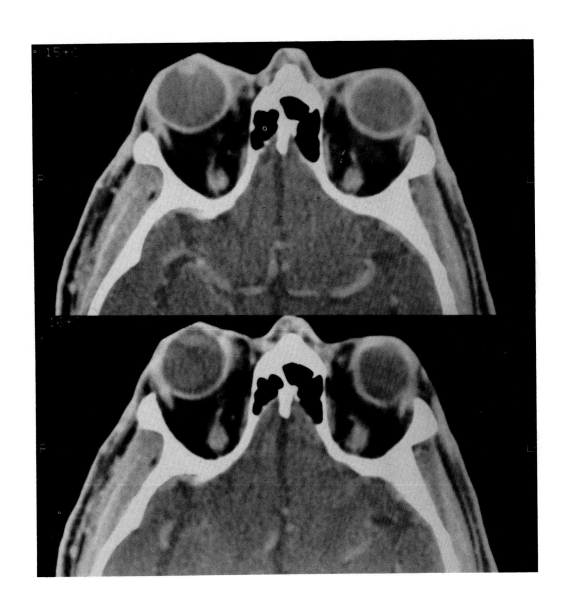

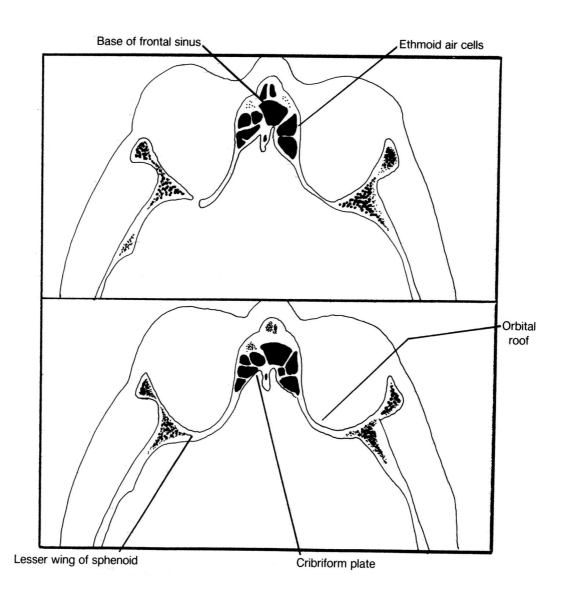

Base of frontal sinus

Ethmoid air cells

Orbital roof

Lesser wing of sphenoid

Cribriform plate

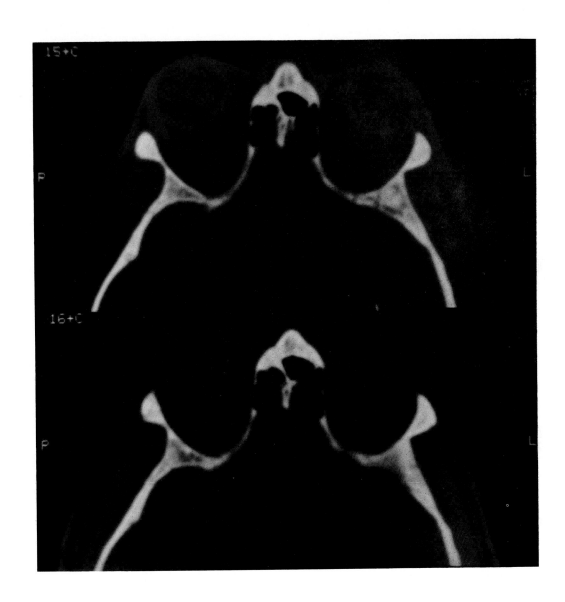

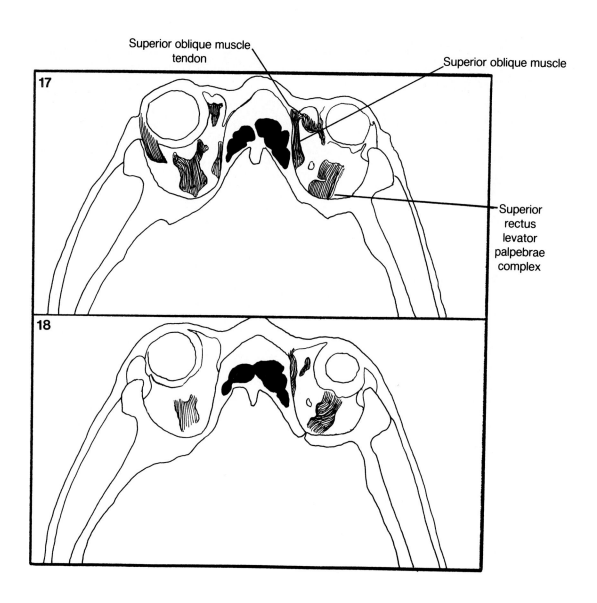

Superior oblique muscle
tendon

Superior oblique muscle

Superior
rectus
levator
palpebrae
complex

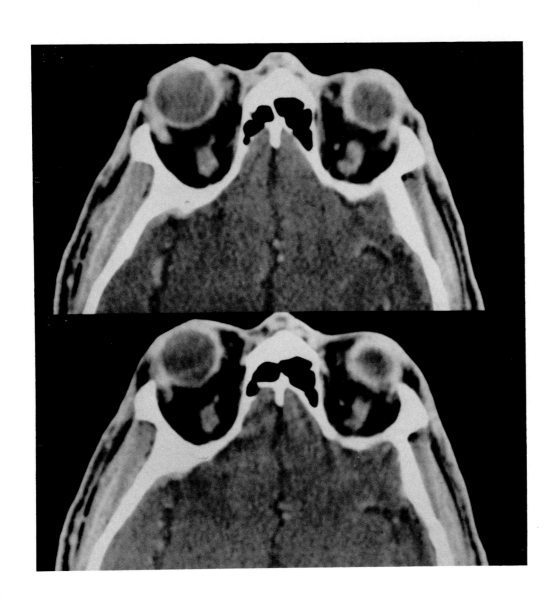

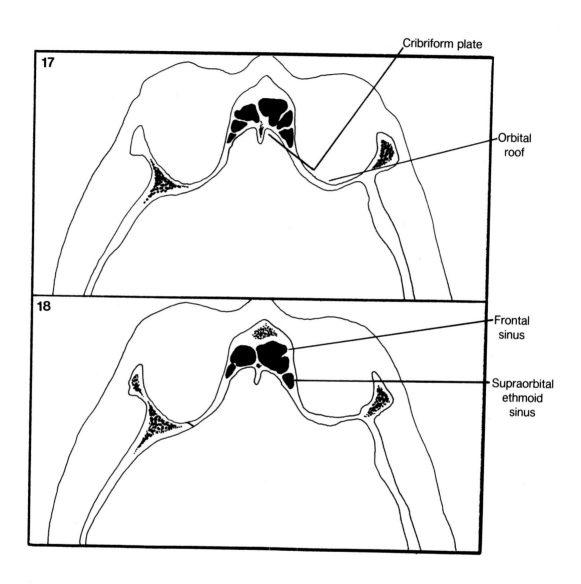

Cribriform plate

Orbital roof

Frontal sinus

Supraorbital ethmoid sinus

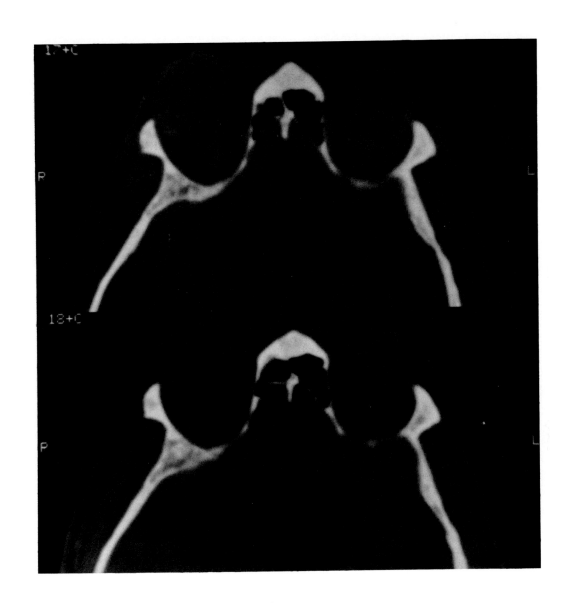

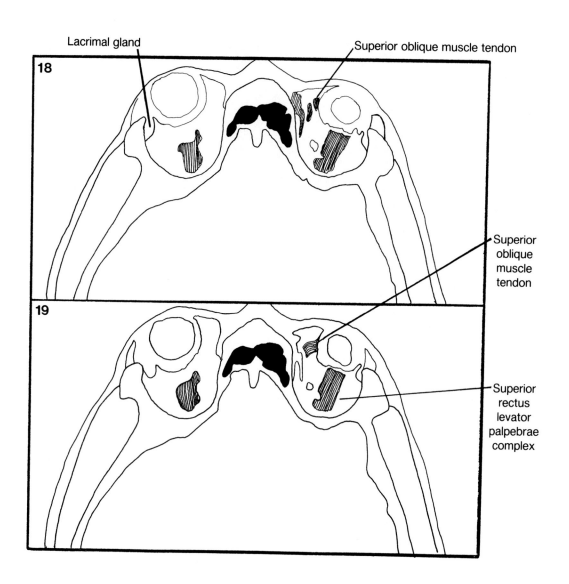

Lacrimal gland

Superior oblique muscle tendon

18

Superior
oblique
muscle
tendon

19

Superior
rectus
levator
palpebrae
complex

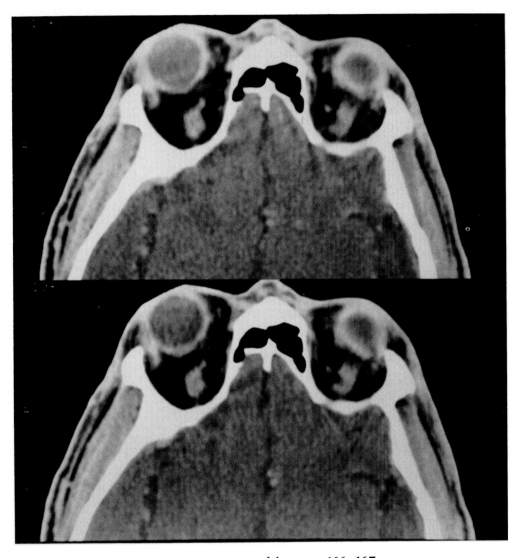

Image 18 is repeated from pp 166, 167.

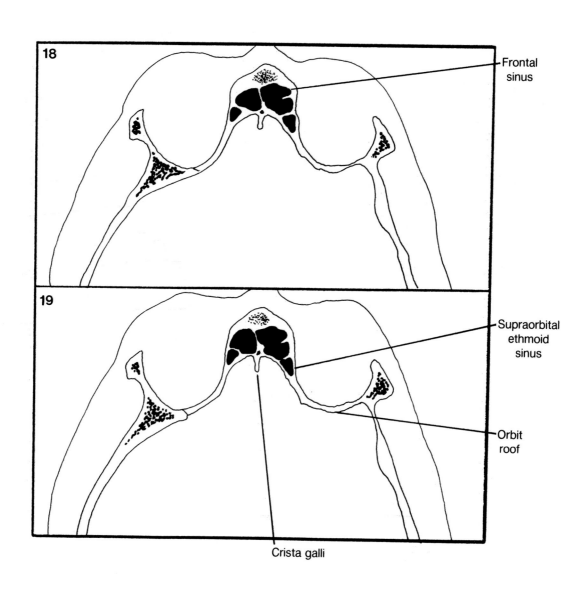

18 — Frontal sinus

19 — Supraorbital ethmoid sinus

— Orbit roof

Crista galli

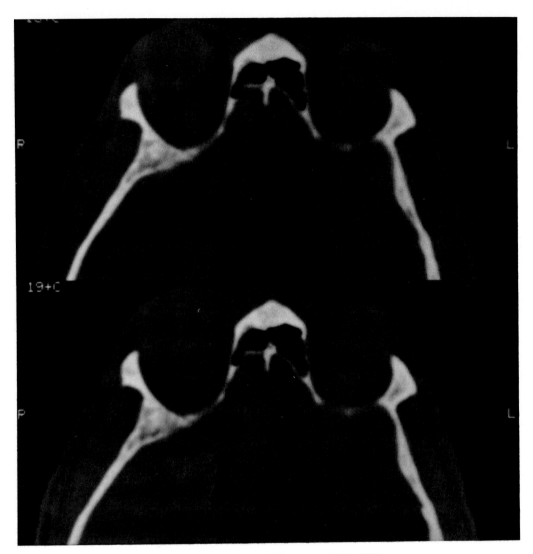

Image 18 is repeated from pp 166, 167.

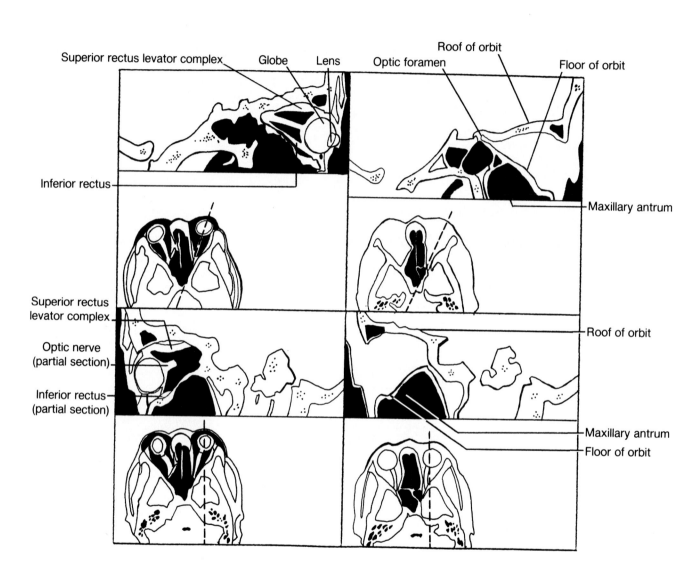

Superior rectus levator complex
Globe
Lens
Optic foramen
Roof of orbit
Floor of orbit

Inferior rectus

Maxillary antrum

Superior rectus
levator complex

Optic nerve
(partial section)

Roof of orbit

Inferior rectus
(partial section)

Maxillary antrum
Floor of orbit

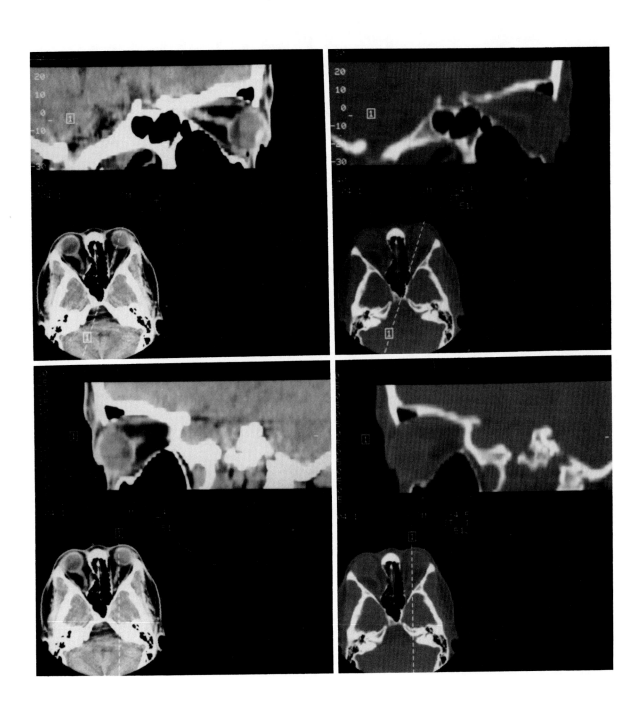

4 Paranasal Sinuses and Naso-pharynx

Axial CT images of the paranasal sinuses and nasopharynx are routinely obtained in a plane parallel to Reid's base line or to the hard palate. The area extending from below the hard palate through the frontal sinuses should be scanned. When patient positioning permits, direct coronal scans of the area from the maxilla antra through the sphenoidal sinuses are recommended. Coronal scans may be performed with the patient in the prone position or supine ("hanging head") position. Both soft tissue and bone window settings are essential. Scan sections are generally 5 mm thick and obtained at 5-mm intervals, although thinner sections may be used as considered necessary. Because these sections necessarily pass through the orbits, some orbital details are included. Soft tissue and bone window images are presented in both the sagittal and coronal planes.

Paranasal Sinuses and Nasopharynx: Axial Plane without Intravenous Contrast

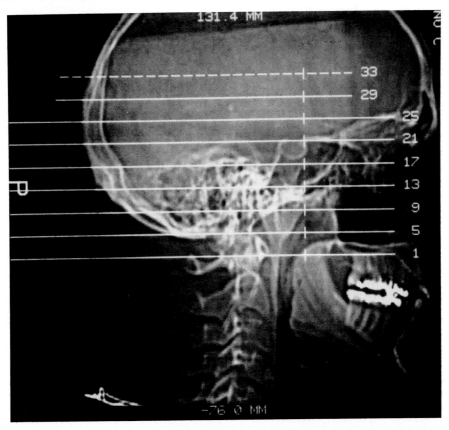

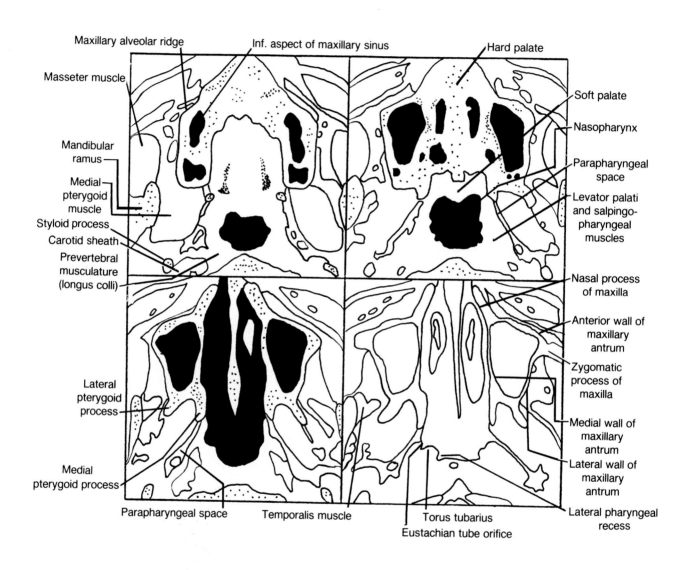

Maxillary alveolar ridge

Inf. aspect of maxillary sinus

Hard palate

Masseter muscle

Soft palate

Nasopharynx

Mandibular ramus

Parapharyngeal space

Medial pterygoid muscle

Levator palati and salpingopharyngeal muscles

Styloid process

Carotid sheath

Prevertebral musculature (longus colli)

Nasal process of maxilla

Anterior wall of maxillary antrum

Zygomatic process of maxilla

Lateral pterygoid process

Medial wall of maxillary antrum

Lateral wall of maxillary antrum

Medial pterygoid process

Parapharyngeal space

Temporalis muscle

Torus tubarius

Eustachian tube orifice

Lateral pharyngeal recess

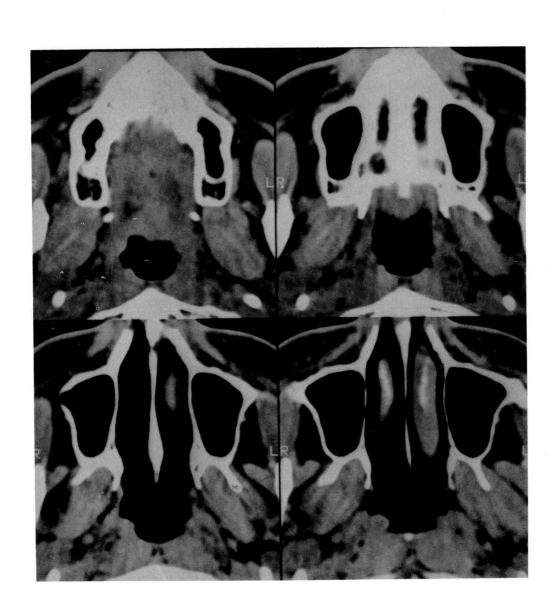

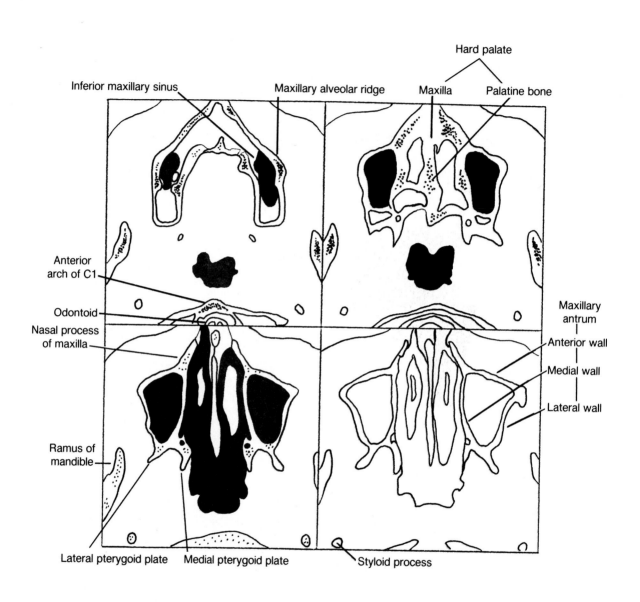

Inferior maxillary sinus

Maxillary alveolar ridge

Hard palate

Maxilla   Palatine bone

Anterior arch of C1

Odontoid

Nasal process of maxilla

Ramus of mandible

Maxillary antrum

Anterior wall

Medial wall

Lateral wall

Lateral pterygoid plate   Medial pterygoid plate

Styloid process

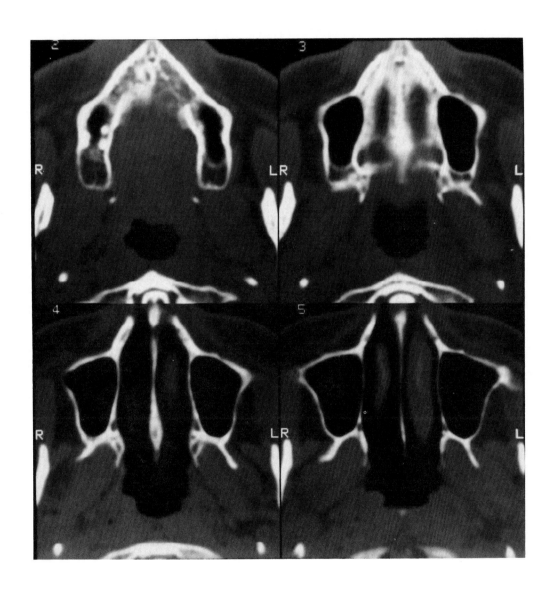

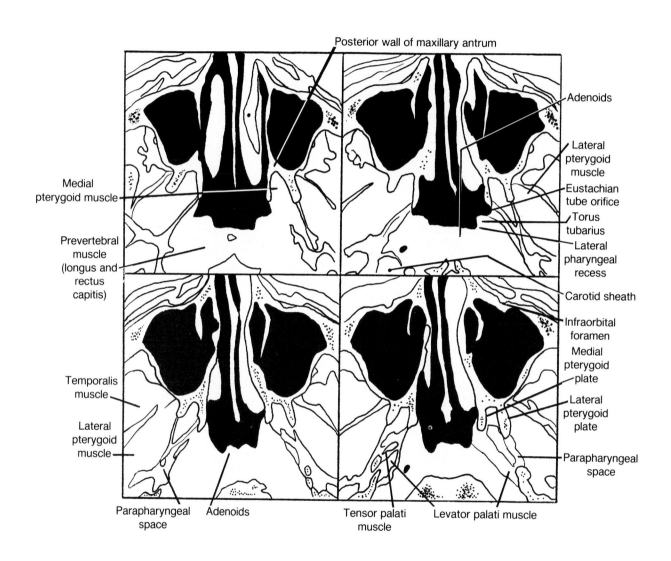

Posterior wall of maxillary antrum

Adenoids

Lateral pterygoid muscle

Eustachian tube orifice

Torus tubarius

Lateral pharyngeal recess

Carotid sheath

Infraorbital foramen

Medial pterygoid plate

Lateral pterygoid plate

Parapharyngeal space

Medial pterygoid muscle

Prevertebral muscle (longus and rectus capitis)

Temporalis muscle

Lateral pterygoid muscle

Parapharyngeal space

Adenoids

Tensor palati muscle

Levator palati muscle

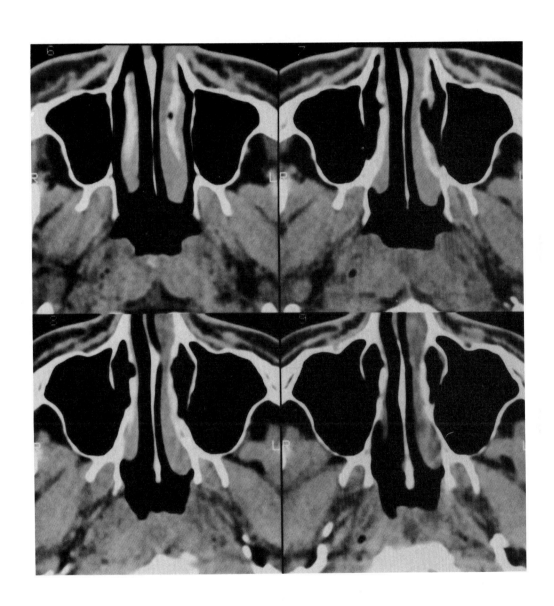

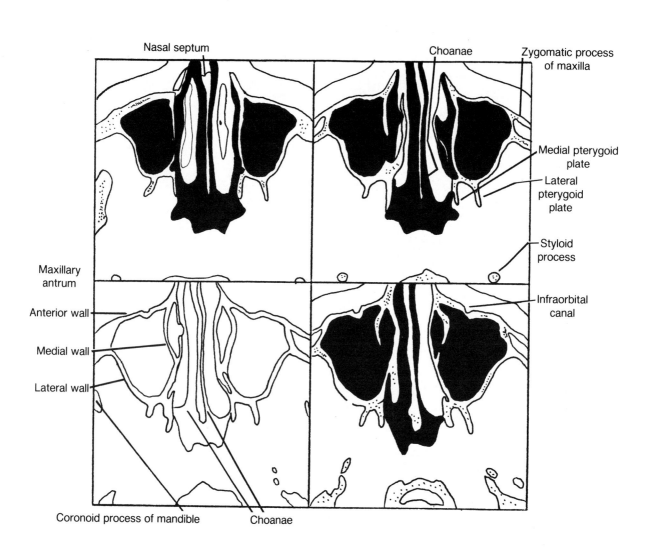

Nasal septum

Choanae

Zygomatic process of maxilla

Medial pterygoid plate

Lateral pterygoid plate

Styloid process

Maxillary antrum

Anterior wall

Medial wall

Lateral wall

Infraorbital canal

Coronoid process of mandible

Choanae

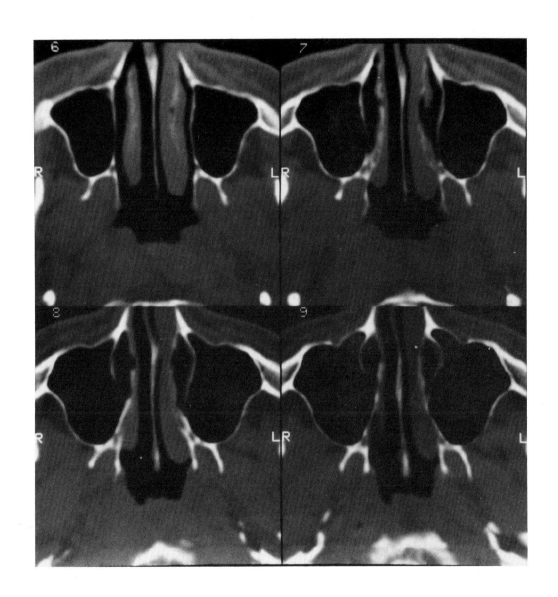

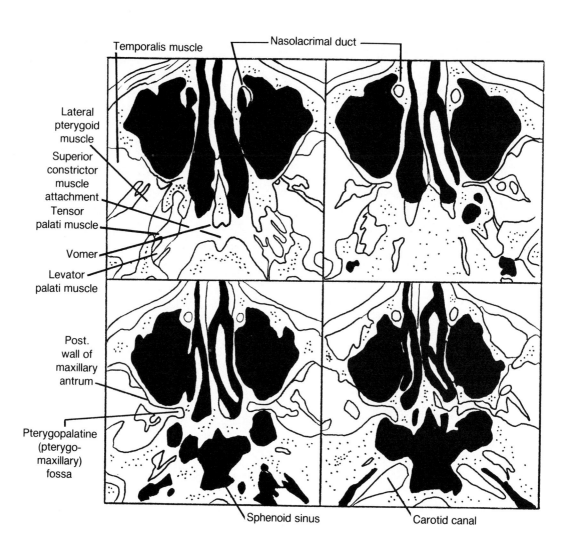

Temporalis muscle

Nasolacrimal duct

Lateral pterygoid muscle

Superior constrictor muscle attachment

Tensor palati muscle

Vomer

Levator palati muscle

Post. wall of maxillary antrum

Pterygopalatine (pterygomaxillary) fossa

Sphenoid sinus

Carotid canal

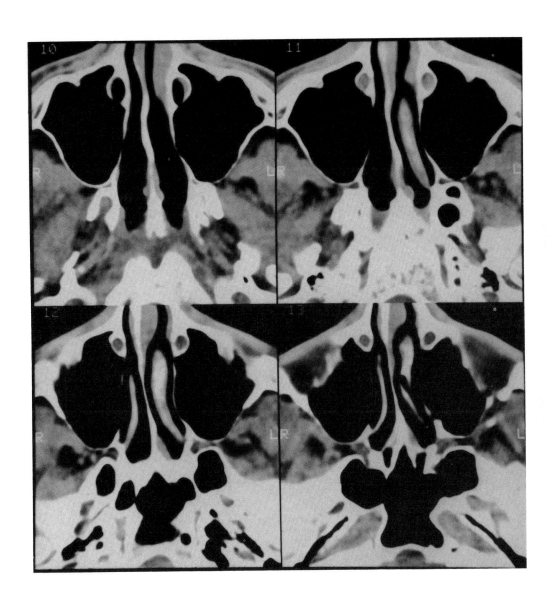

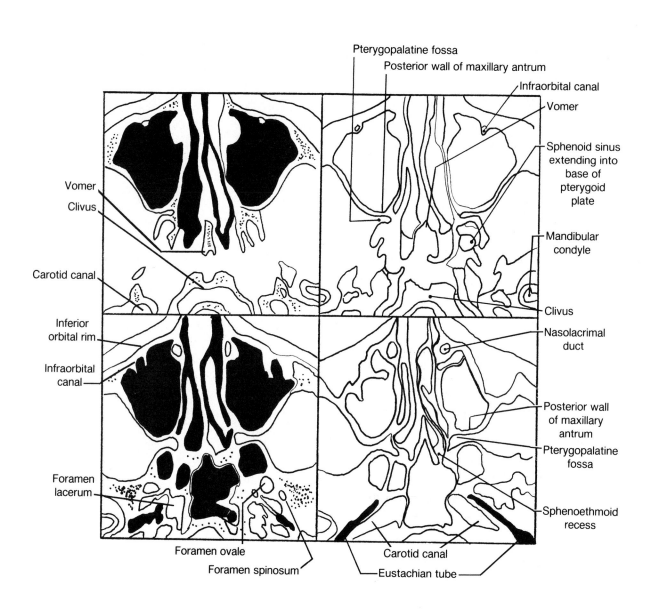

Pterygopalatine fossa

Posterior wall of maxillary antrum

Infraorbital canal

Vomer

Sphenoid sinus extending into base of pterygoid plate

Mandibular condyle

Clivus

Nasolacrimal duct

Posterior wall of maxillary antrum

Pterygopalatine fossa

Sphenoethmoid recess

Vomer

Clivus

Carotid canal

Inferior orbital rim

Infraorbital canal

Foramen lacerum

Foramen ovale

Foramen spinosum

Carotid canal

Eustachian tube

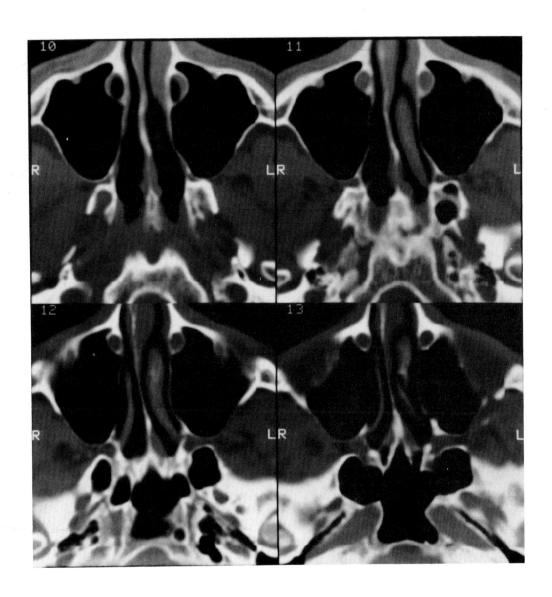

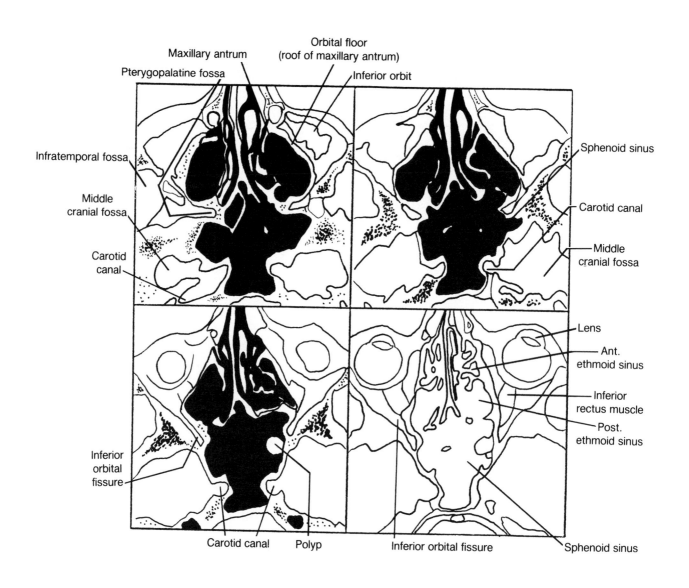

Pterygopalatine fossa

Maxillary antrum

Orbital floor
(roof of maxillary antrum)

Inferior orbit

Infratemporal fossa

Middle
cranial fossa

Carotid
canal

Sphenoid sinus

Carotid canal

Middle
cranial fossa

Inferior
orbital
fissure

Lens

Ant.
ethmoid sinus

Inferior
rectus muscle

Post.
ethmoid sinus

Carotid canal   Polyp

Inferior orbital fissure

Sphenoid sinus

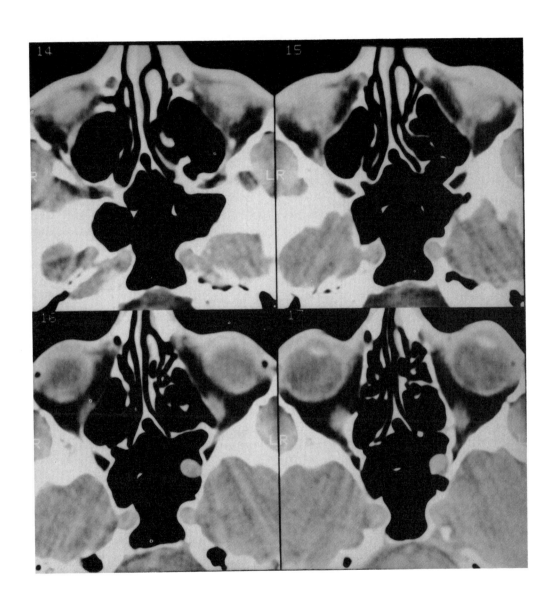

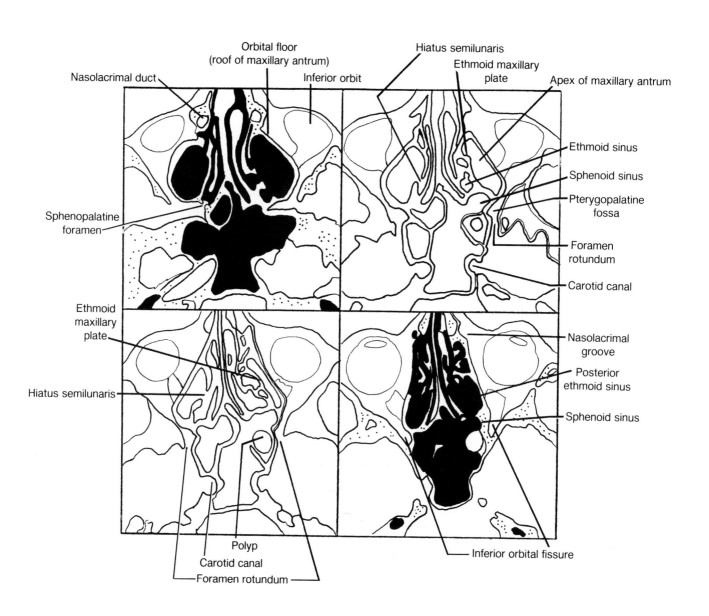

Nasolacrimal duct

Orbital floor
(roof of maxillary antrum)

Inferior orbit

Hiatus semilunaris

Ethmoid maxillary
plate

Apex of maxillary antrum

Ethmoid sinus

Sphenoid sinus

Pterygopalatine
fossa

Foramen
rotundum

Carotid canal

Sphenopalatine
foramen

Ethmoid
maxillary
plate

Hiatus semilunaris

Nasolacrimal
groove

Posterior
ethmoid sinus

Sphenoid sinus

Polyp

Carotid canal

Foramen rotundum

Inferior orbital fissure

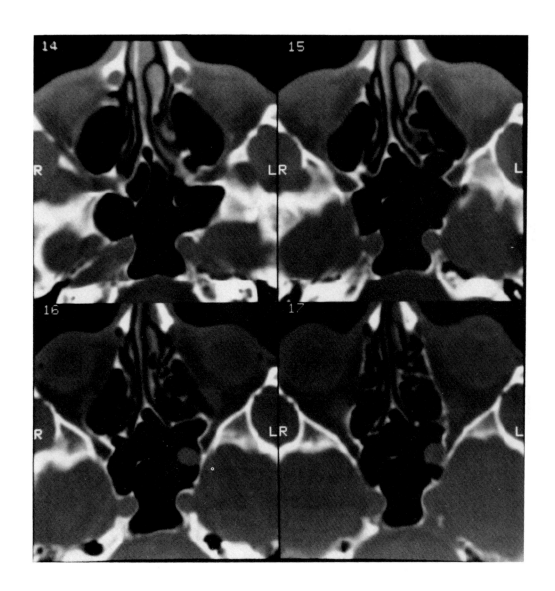

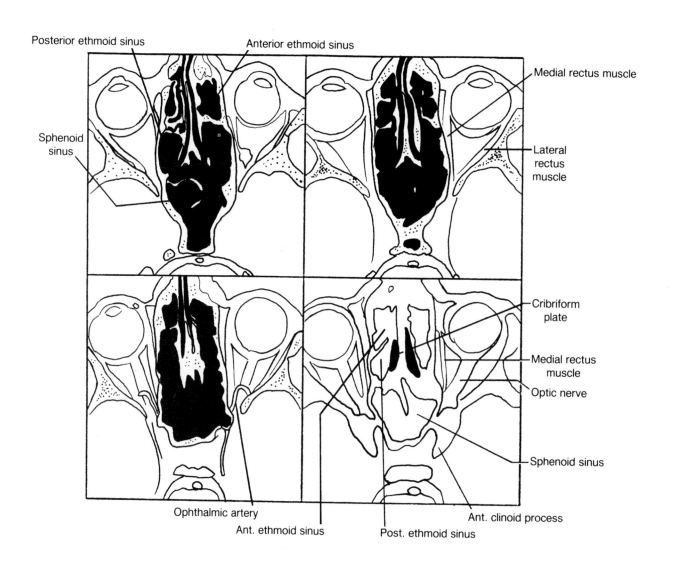

Posterior ethmoid sinus

Anterior ethmoid sinus

Medial rectus muscle

Sphenoid sinus

Lateral rectus muscle

Cribriform plate

Medial rectus muscle

Optic nerve

Sphenoid sinus

Ophthalmic artery

Ant. ethmoid sinus

Post. ethmoid sinus

Ant. clinoid process

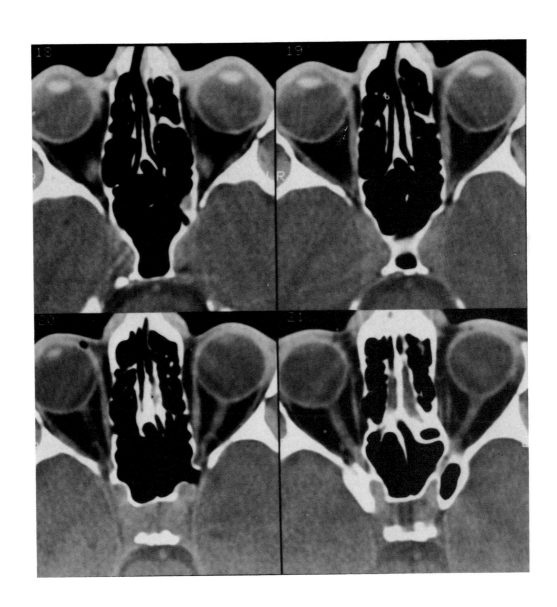

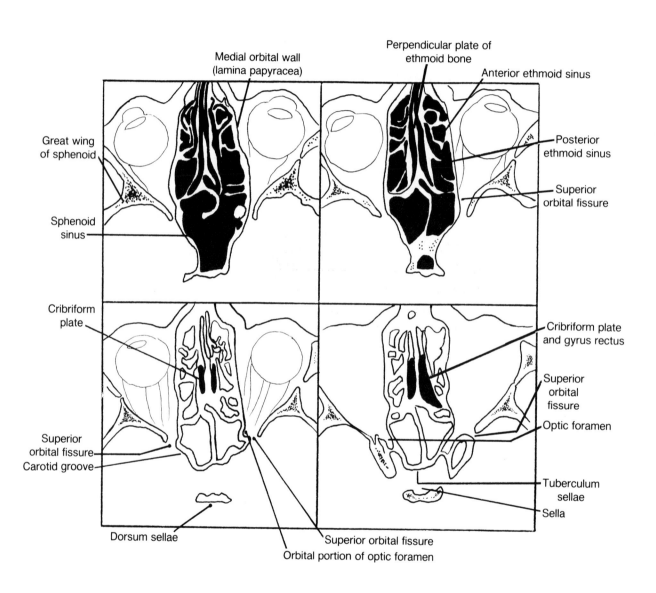

Medial orbital wall
(lamina papyracea)

Perpendicular plate of
ethmoid bone

Anterior ethmoid sinus

Great wing
of sphenoid

Sphenoid
sinus

Posterior
ethmoid sinus

Superior
orbital fissure

Cribriform
plate

Cribriform plate
and gyrus rectus

Superior
orbital
fissure

Optic foramen

Superior
orbital fissure

Carotid groove

Tuberculum
sellae

Sella

Dorsum sellae

Superior orbital fissure

Orbital portion of optic foramen

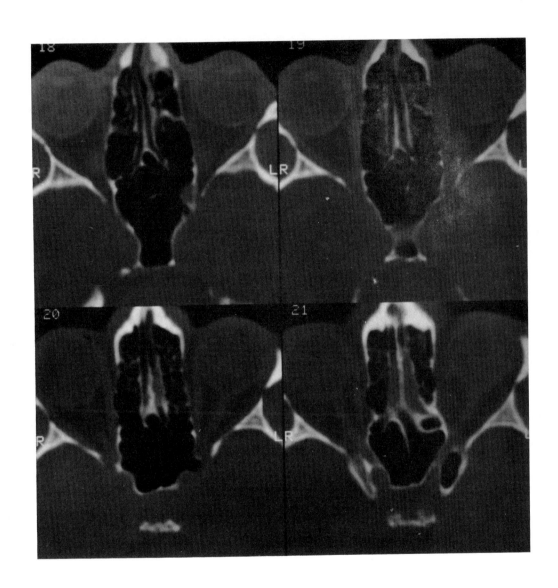

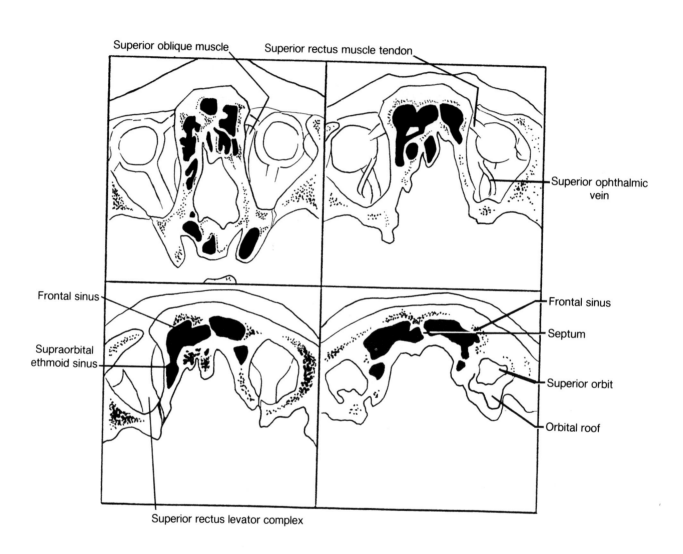

Superior oblique muscle

Superior rectus muscle tendon

Superior ophthalmic vein

Frontal sinus

Supraorbital ethmoid sinus

Frontal sinus

Septum

Superior orbit

Orbital roof

Superior rectus levator complex

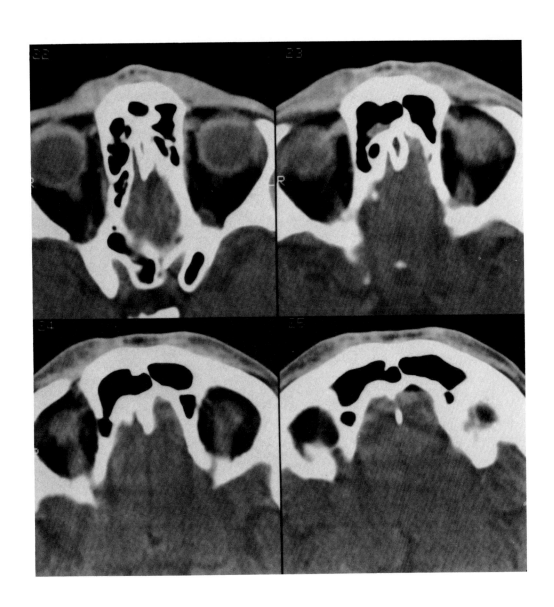

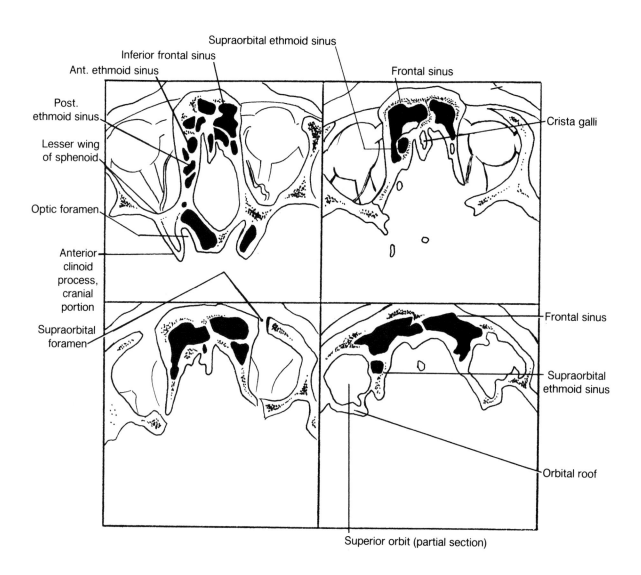

Supraorbital ethmoid sinus

Inferior frontal sinus

Ant. ethmoid sinus

Frontal sinus

Post. ethmoid sinus

Lesser wing of sphenoid

Crista galli

Optic foramen

Anterior clinoid process, cranial portion

Supraorbital foramen

Frontal sinus

Supraorbital ethmoid sinus

Orbital roof

Superior orbit (partial section)

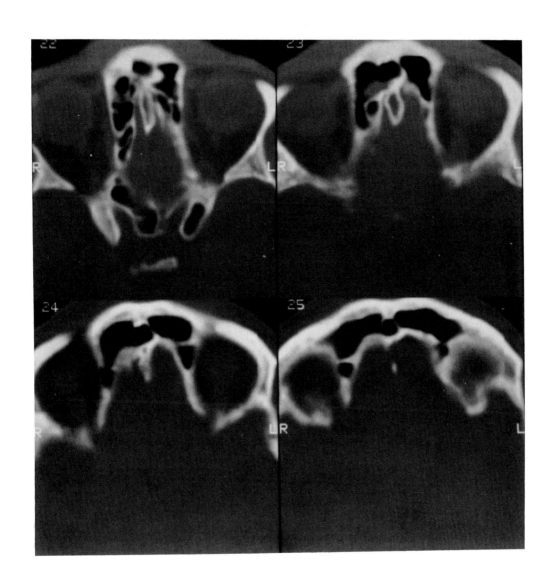

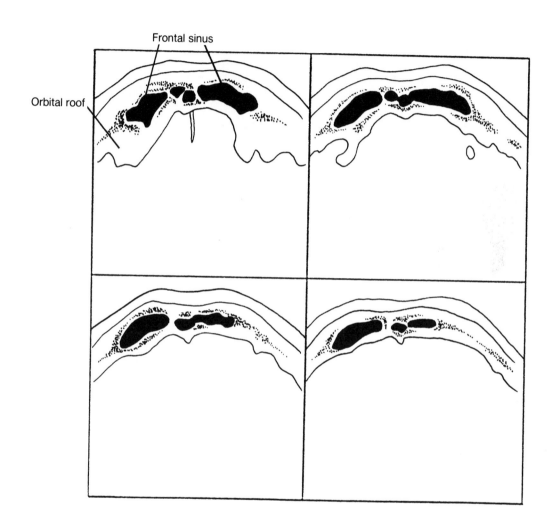

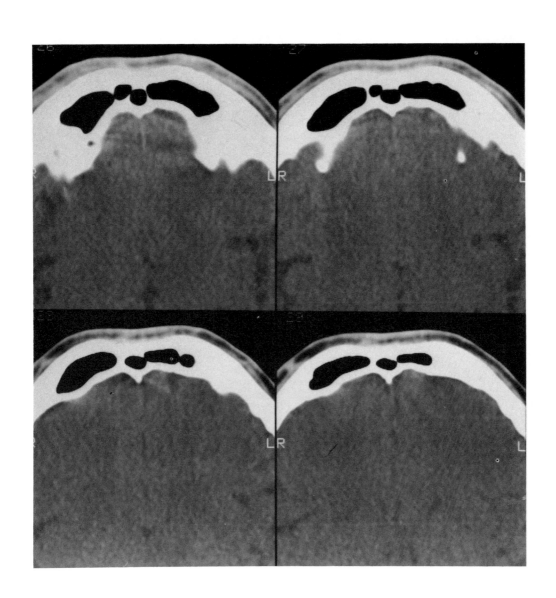

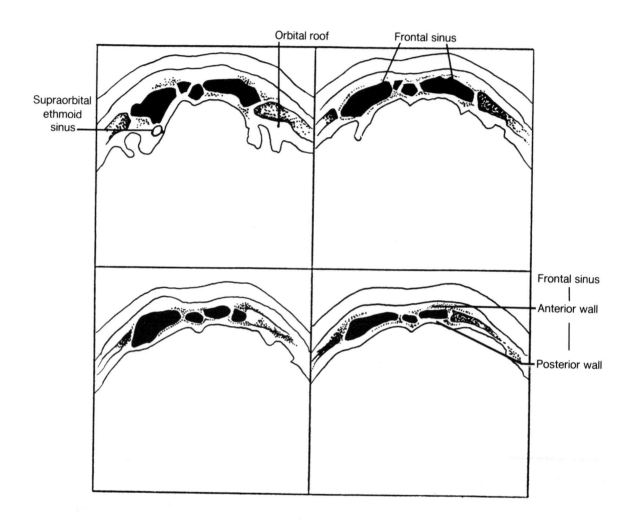

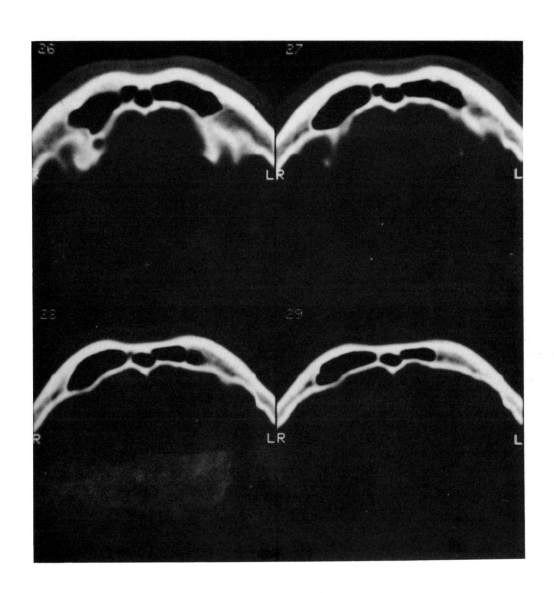

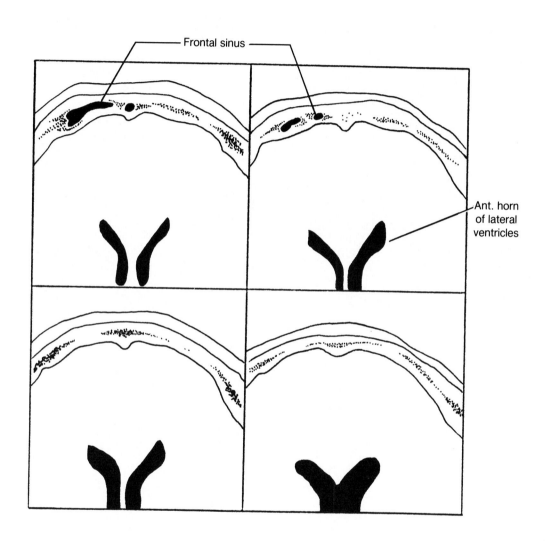

Frontal sinus

Ant. horn
of lateral
ventricles

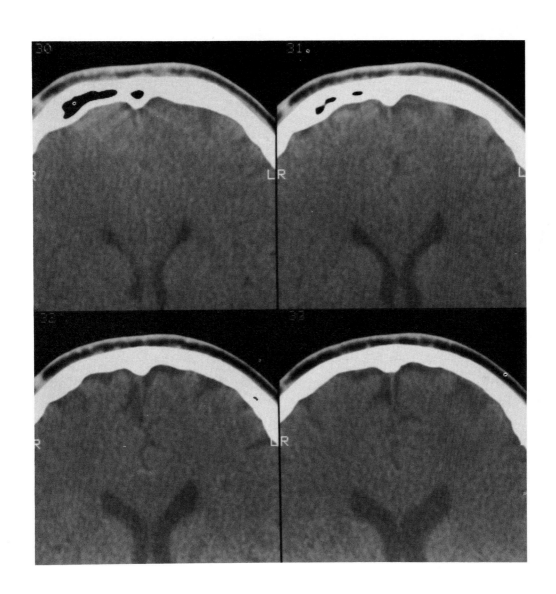

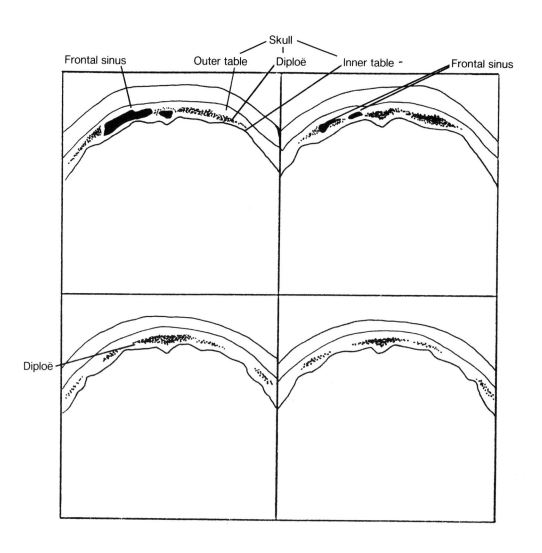

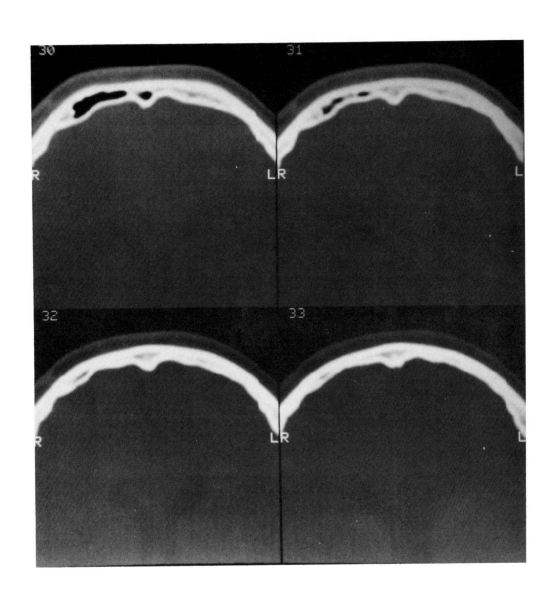

Paranasal Sinuses and Nasopharynx: Coronal Plane with Intravenous Contrast

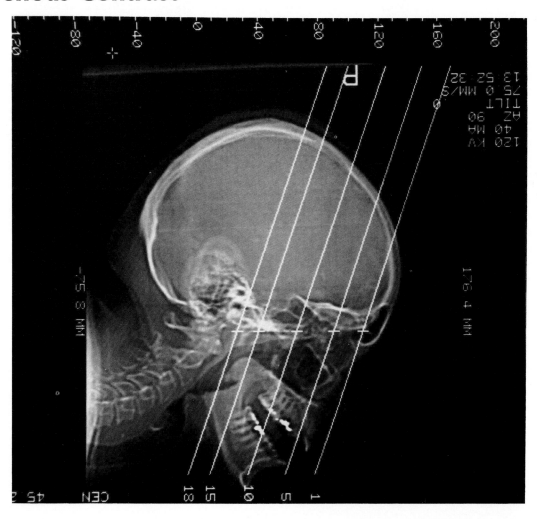

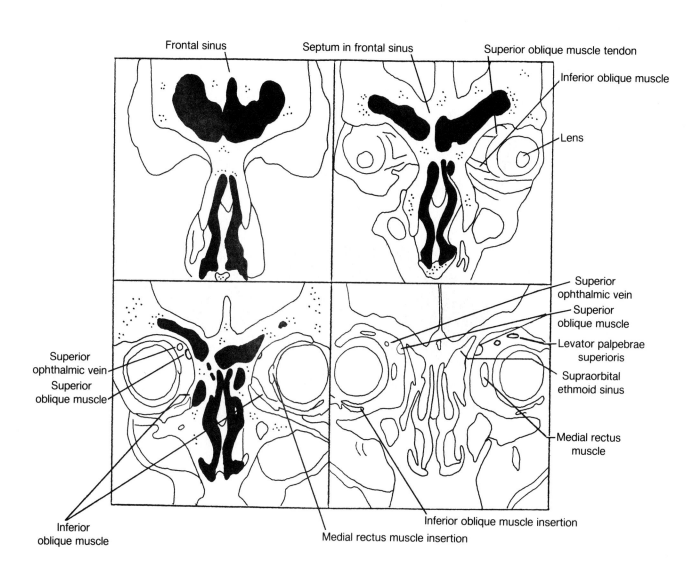

Frontal sinus

Septum in frontal sinus

Superior oblique muscle tendon

Inferior oblique muscle

Lens

Superior
ophthalmic vein

Superior
oblique muscle

Levator palpebrae
superioris

Supraorbital
ethmoid sinus

Medial rectus
muscle

Superior
ophthalmic vein

Superior
oblique muscle

Inferior
oblique muscle

Medial rectus muscle insertion

Inferior oblique muscle insertion

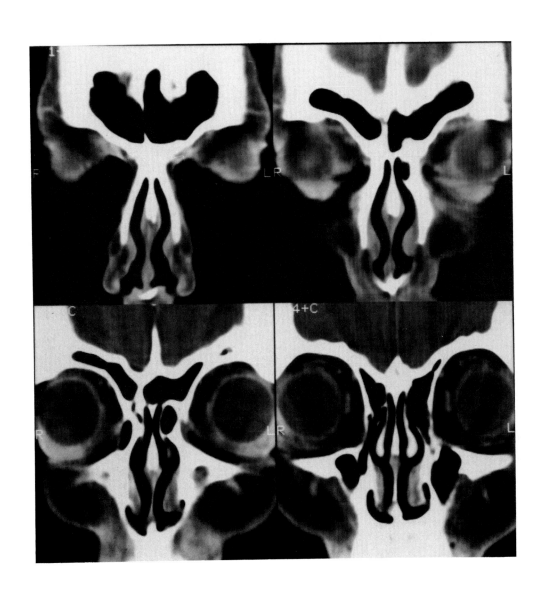

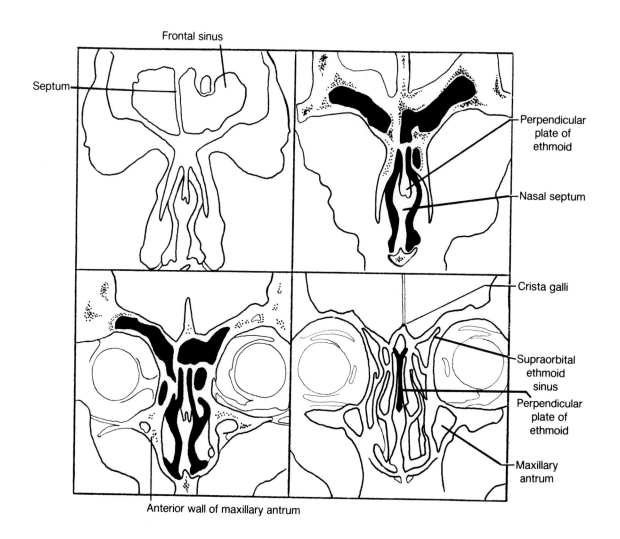

Frontal sinus

Septum

Perpendicular
plate of
ethmoid

Nasal septum

Crista galli

Supraorbital
ethmoid
sinus

Perpendicular
plate of
ethmoid

Maxillary
antrum

Anterior wall of maxillary antrum

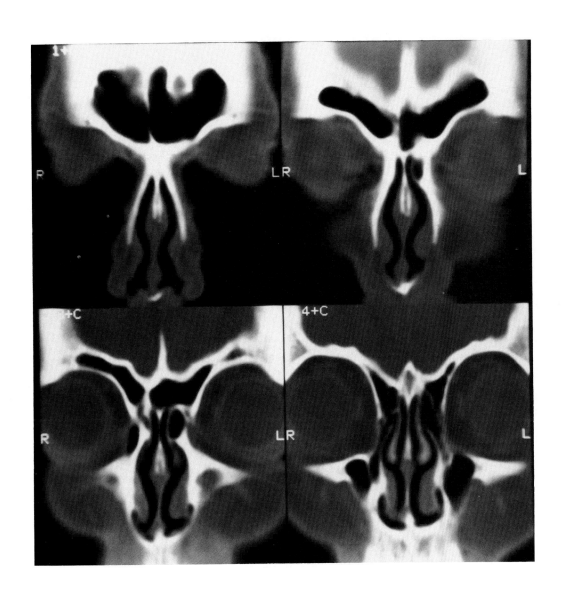

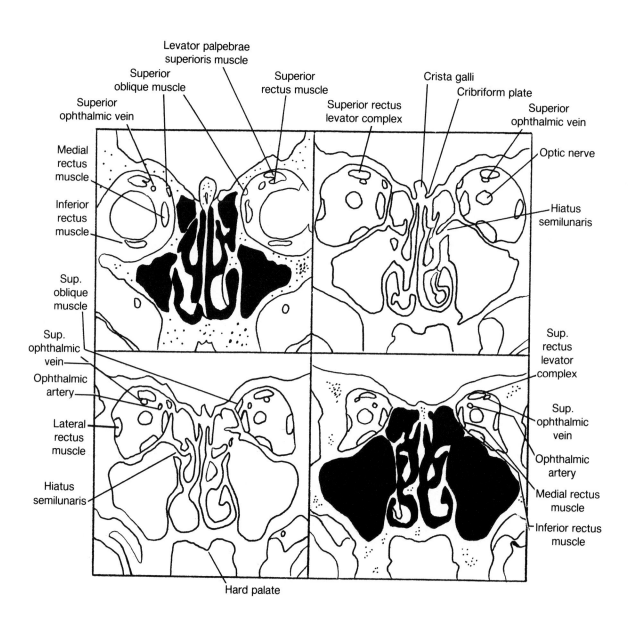

Levator palpebrae
superioris muscle

Superior
oblique muscle

Superior
ophthalmic vein

Superior
rectus muscle

Superior rectus
levator complex

Crista galli

Cribriform plate

Superior
ophthalmic vein

Optic nerve

Medial
rectus
muscle

Inferior
rectus
muscle

Hiatus
semilunaris

Sup.
oblique
muscle

Sup.
rectus
levator
complex

Sup.
ophthalmic
vein

Ophthalmic
artery

Sup.
ophthalmic
vein

Lateral
rectus
muscle

Ophthalmic
artery

Medial rectus
muscle

Hiatus
semilunaris

Inferior rectus
muscle

Hard palate

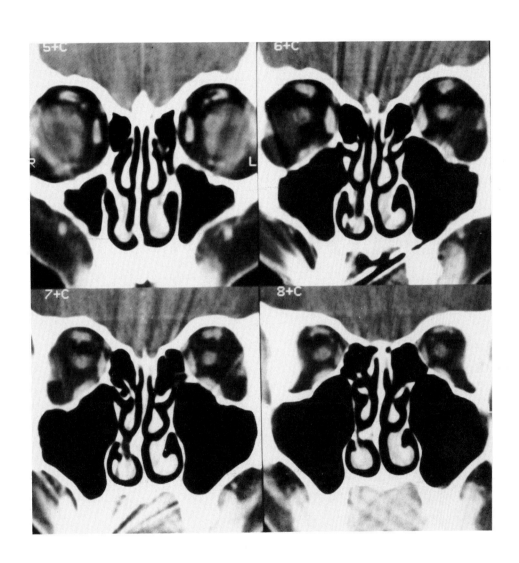

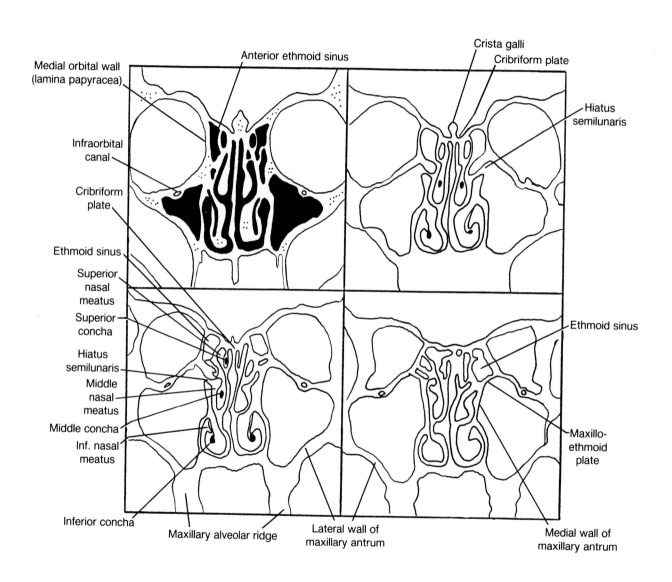

Medial orbital wall (lamina papyracea)

Anterior ethmoid sinus

Crista galli
Cribriform plate

Hiatus semilunaris

Infraorbital canal

Cribriform plate

Ethmoid sinus

Superior nasal meatus

Superior concha

Hiatus semilunaris

Middle nasal meatus

Middle concha

Inf. nasal meatus

Ethmoid sinus

Maxillo-ethmoid plate

Inferior concha

Maxillary alveolar ridge

Lateral wall of maxillary antrum

Medial wall of maxillary antrum

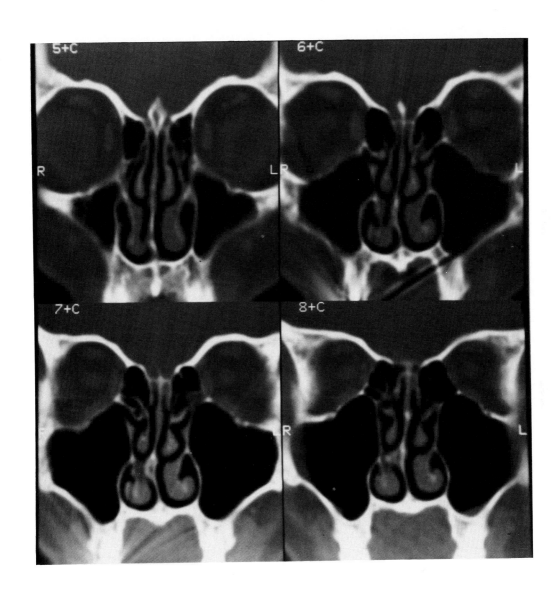

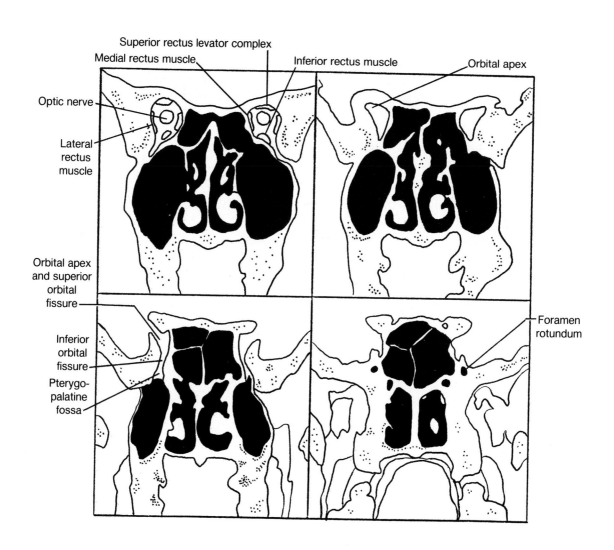

Superior rectus levator complex

Medial rectus muscle

Inferior rectus muscle

Orbital apex

Optic nerve

Lateral rectus muscle

Orbital apex and superior orbital fissure

Inferior orbital fissure

Pterygopalatine fossa

Foramen rotundum

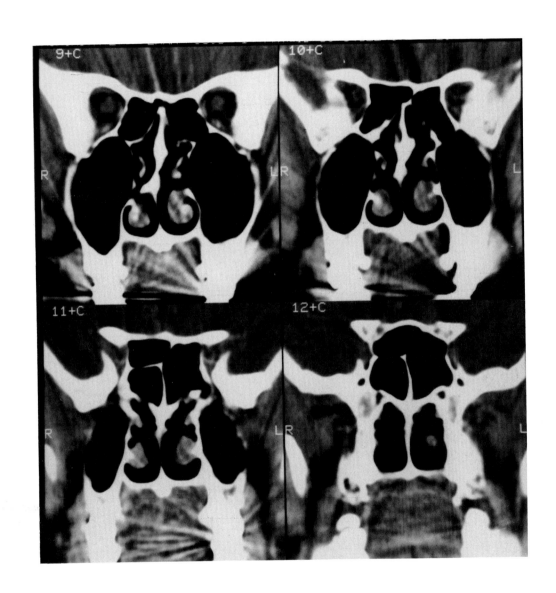

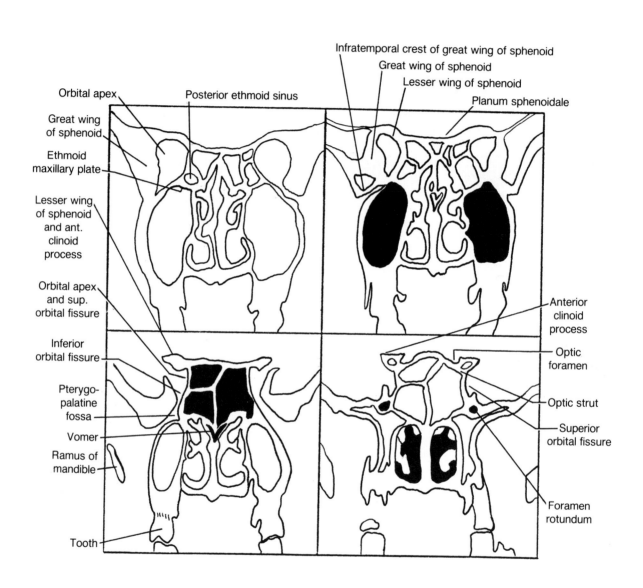

Orbital apex

Great wing
of sphenoid

Ethmoid
maxillary plate

Lesser wing
of sphenoid
and ant.
clinoid
process

Orbital apex
and sup.
orbital fissure

Inferior
orbital fissure

Pterygo-
palatine
fossa

Vomer

Ramus of
mandible

Tooth

Posterior ethmoid sinus

Infratemporal crest of great wing of sphenoid
Great wing of sphenoid
Lesser wing of sphenoid
Planum sphenoidale

Anterior
clinoid
process

Optic
foramen

Optic strut

Superior
orbital fissure

Foramen
rotundum

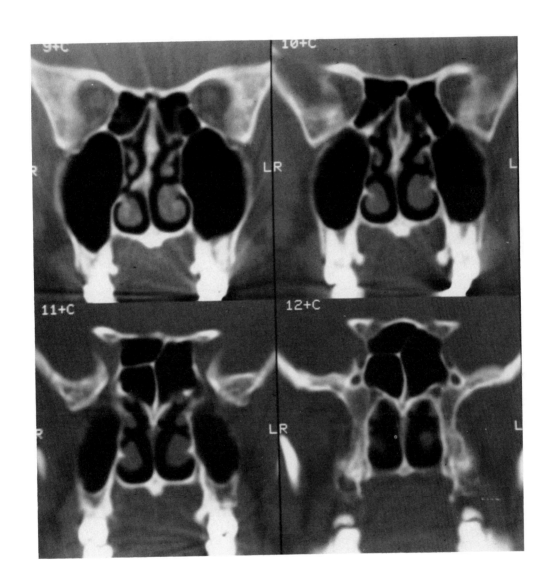

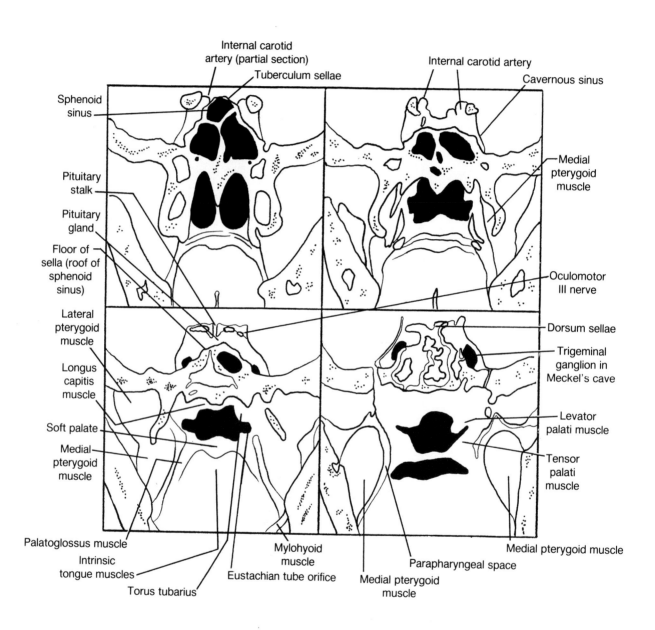

Internal carotid
artery (partial section)

Tuberculum sellae

Internal carotid artery

Cavernous sinus

Sphenoid
sinus

Pituitary
stalk

Pituitary
gland

Floor of
sella (roof of
sphenoid
sinus)

Lateral
pterygoid
muscle

Longus
capitis
muscle

Soft palate

Medial
pterygoid
muscle

Medial
pterygoid
muscle

Oculomotor
III nerve

Dorsum sellae

Trigeminal
ganglion in
Meckel's cave

Levator
palati muscle

Tensor
palati
muscle

Palatoglossus muscle

Intrinsic
tongue muscles

Torus tubarius

Mylohyoid
muscle

Eustachian tube orifice

Medial pterygoid
muscle

Parapharyngeal space

Medial pterygoid muscle

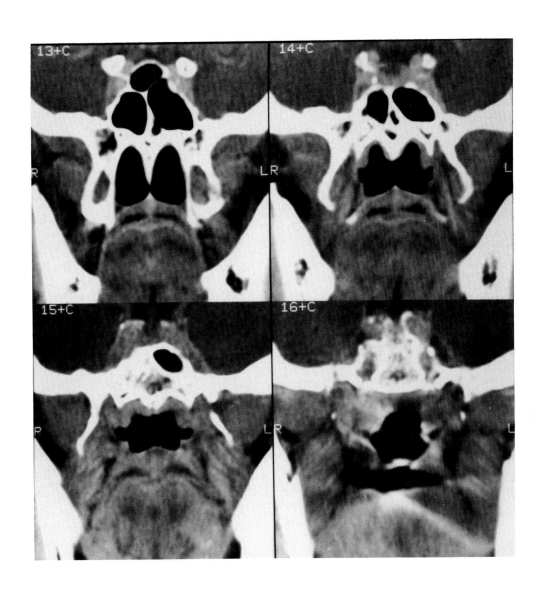

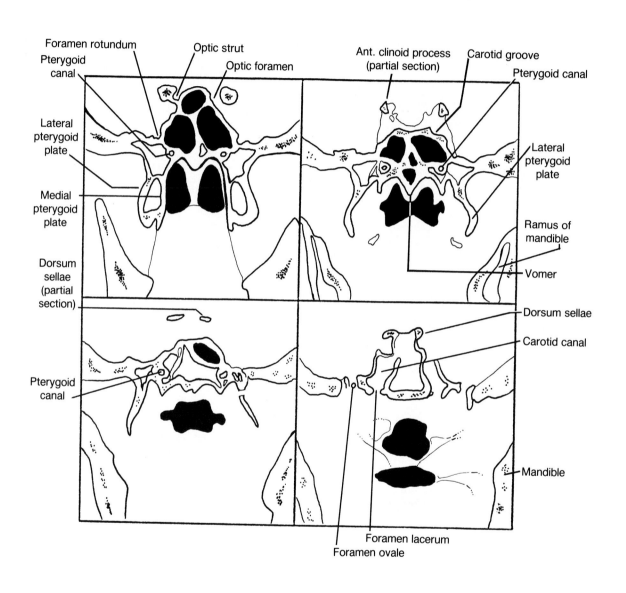

Foramen rotundum
Pterygoid canal
Optic strut
Optic foramen
Ant. clinoid process (partial section)
Carotid groove
Pterygoid canal

Lateral pterygoid plate
Medial pterygoid plate
Lateral pterygoid plate
Ramus of mandible
Vomer

Dorsum sellae (partial section)

Dorsum sellae
Carotid canal

Pterygoid canal

Mandible

Foramen lacerum
Foramen ovale

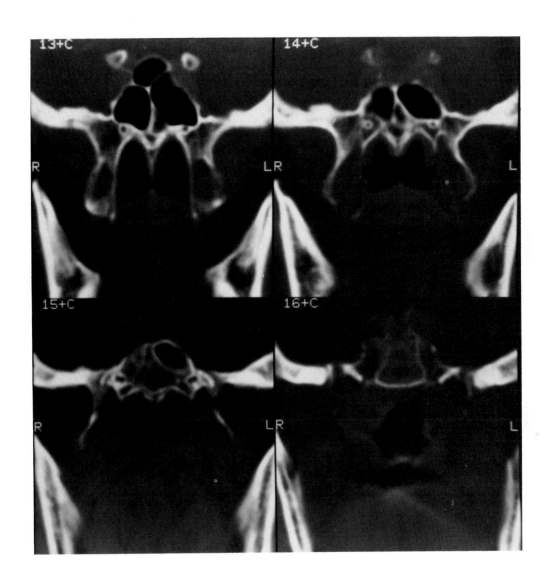

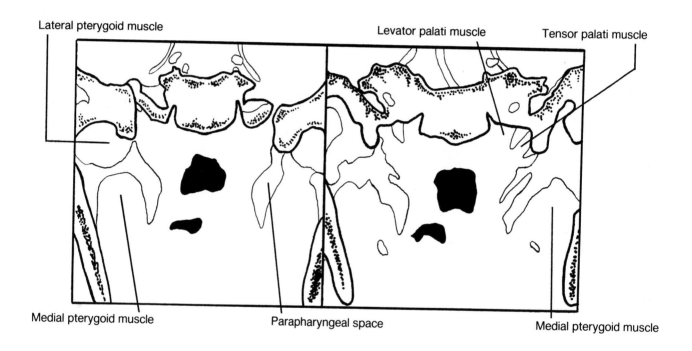

Lateral pterygoid muscle

Levator palati muscle

Tensor palati muscle

Medial pterygoid muscle

Parapharyngeal space

Medial pterygoid muscle

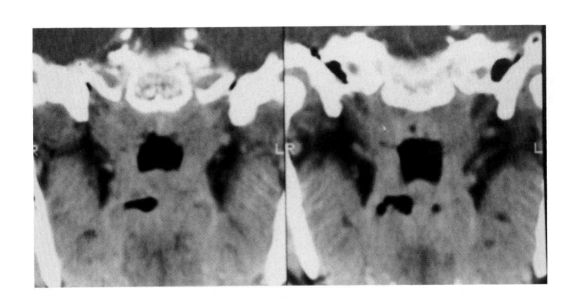

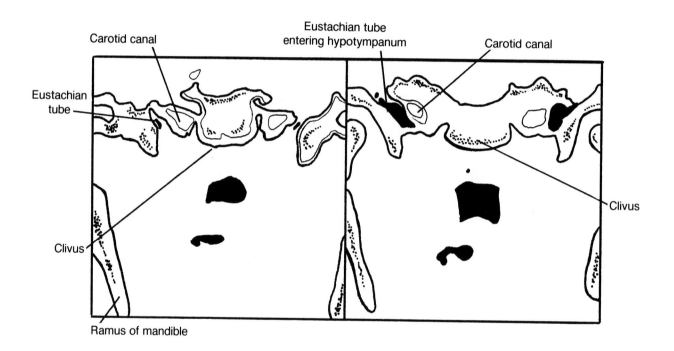

Carotid canal

Eustachian tube entering hypotympanum

Carotid canal

Eustachian tube

Clivus

Clivus

Ramus of mandible

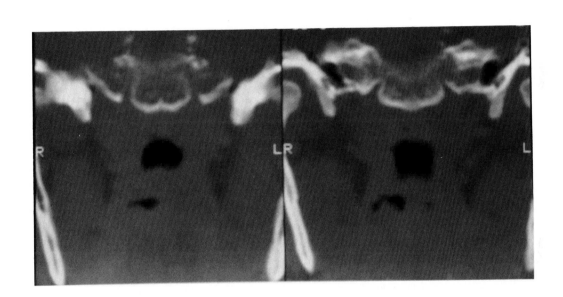

5 Temporal Bone

High-resolution temporal bone scans are performed in axial and coronal planes using 1.5-mm sections, the bone algorithm, and a display field of view of 12.8 on the GE 9800 scanner. The raw data must be saved following the scan for application of this high-resolution technique. X and Y coordinates must be specified on the initial images in order to be used as the center of the expanded images. A large image format was used with multiple display imaging menu to obtain the life-size images shown in this chapter. For the examination of children, or if reformatted images are desired, 1.5-mm sections at 1-mm intervals are recommended.

The axial scan plane used here is +30° to Reid's base line, and extends from the external auditory canal tangent to the orbital roof. The coronal plane is oriented at +105° to Reid's base line and is parallel to the ramus of the mandible. The starting point in each case should be the temporomandibular joint, with consecutive sections obtained until the petrous ridges and mastoid areas are completely delineated. This usually requires about 20 axial and 20 coronal sections. Other scan planes may be used as necessary, depending on the anatomic structures to be defined. As in pituitary scanning, the time required for this examination using the GE 9800 scanner has been dramatically reduced compared to earlier model scanners.

Temporal Bone: Axial Plane

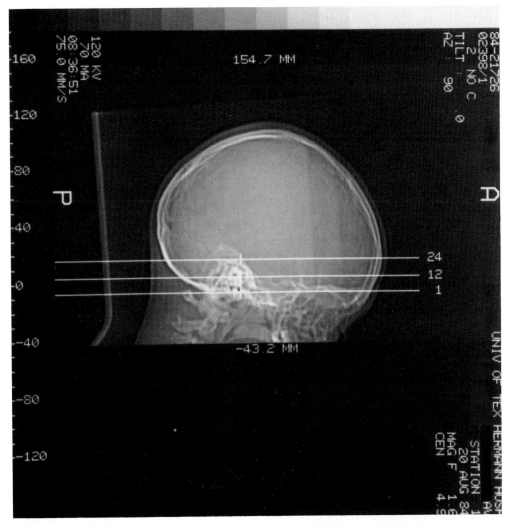

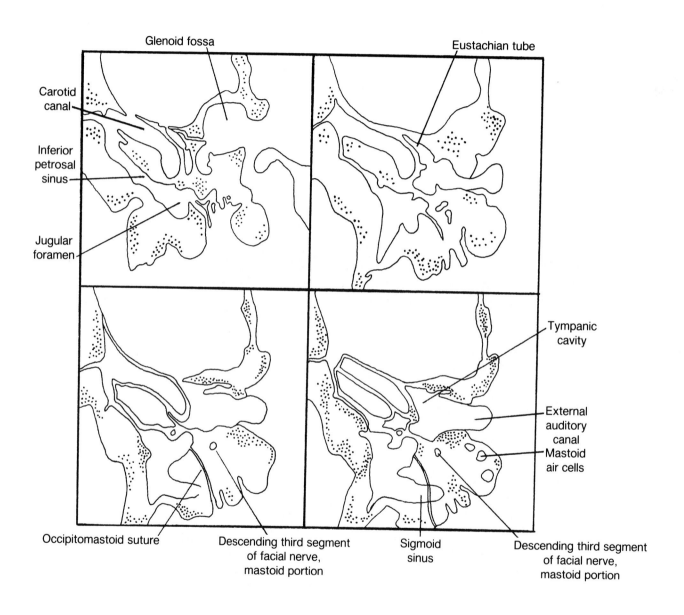

Glenoid fossa

Eustachian tube

Carotid canal

Inferior petrosal sinus

Jugular foramen

Tympanic cavity

External auditory canal

Mastoid air cells

Occipitomastoid suture

Descending third segment of facial nerve, mastoid portion

Sigmoid sinus

Descending third segment of facial nerve, mastoid portion

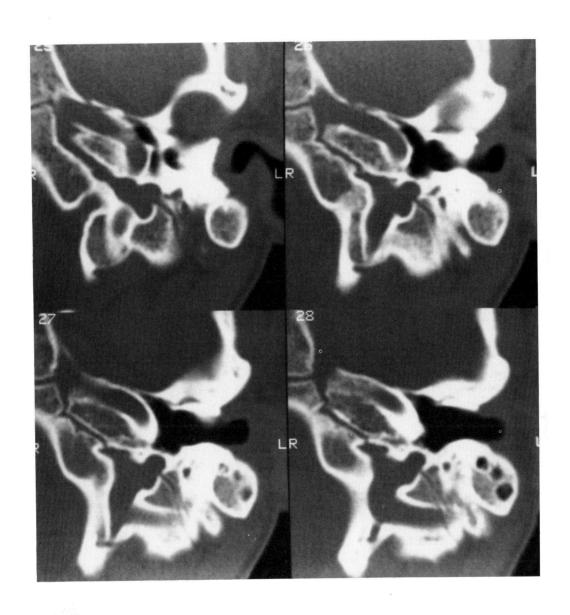

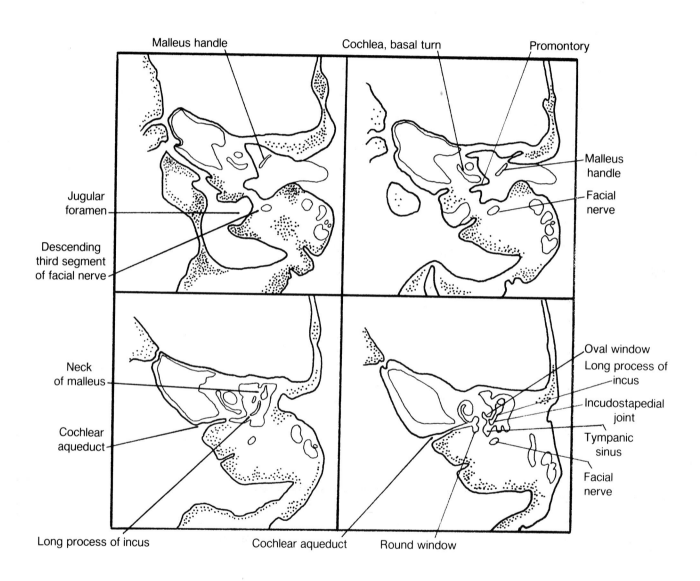

Malleus handle

Cochlea, basal turn

Promontory

Jugular
foramen

Descending
third segment
of facial nerve

Malleus
handle

Facial
nerve

Neck
of malleus

Cochlear
aqueduct

Oval window
Long process of
incus

Incudostapedial
joint

Tympanic
sinus

Facial
nerve

Long process of incus

Cochlear aqueduct

Round window

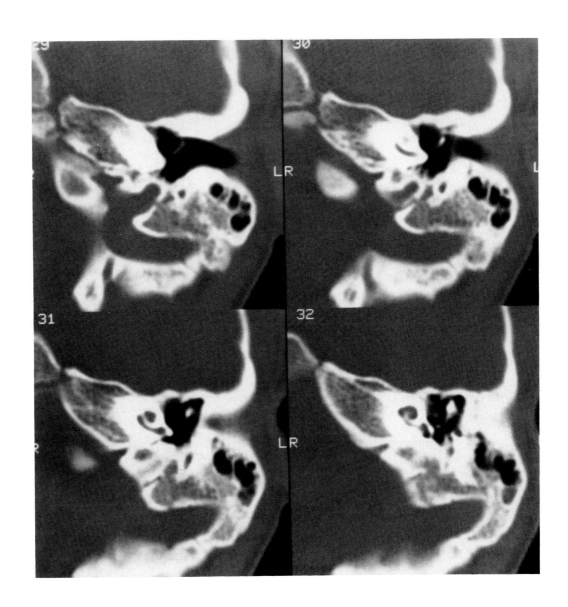

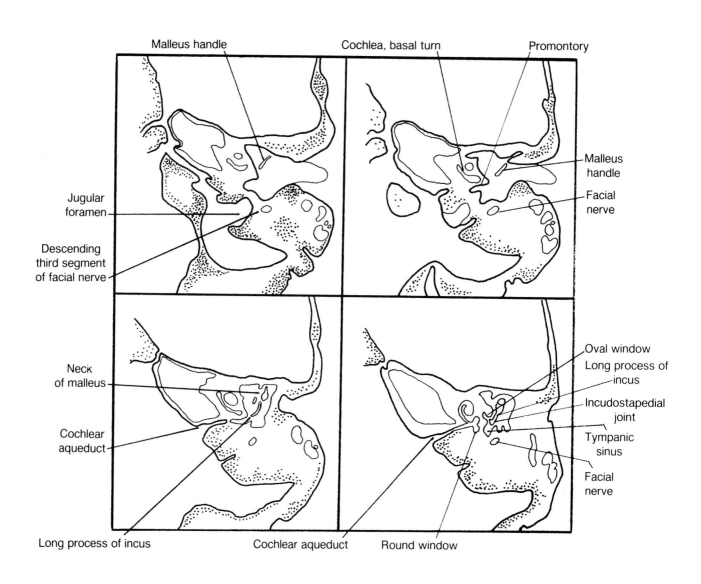

Malleus handle

Cochlea, basal turn

Promontory

Jugular
foramen

Descending
third segment
of facial nerve

Malleus
handle

Facial
nerve

Neck
of malleus

Cochlear
aqueduct

Oval window

Long process of
incus

Incudostapedial
joint

Tympanic
sinus

Facial
nerve

Long process of incus

Cochlear aqueduct

Round window

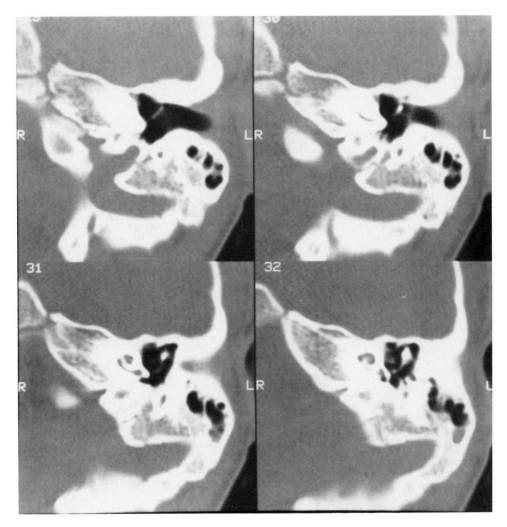

Images 29 through 32 are repeated from p 235 using a lighter photographic technique to emphasize fine detail in the middle ear.

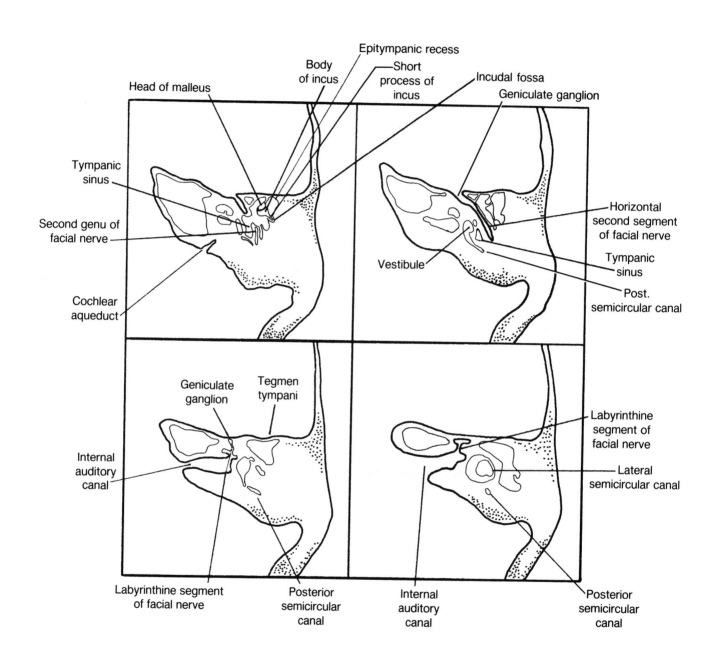

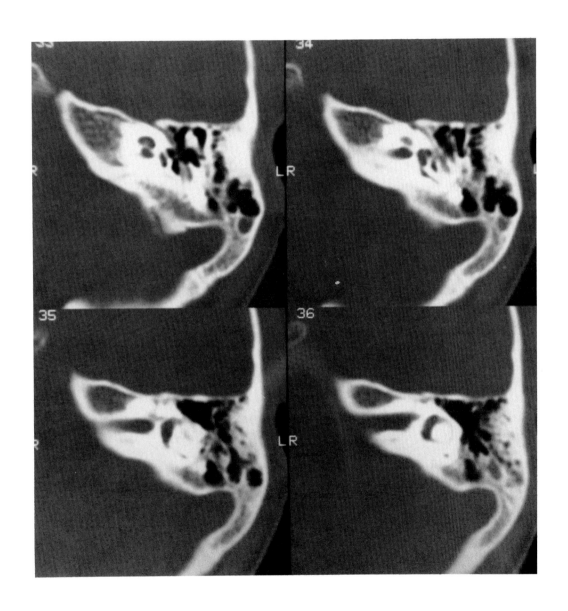

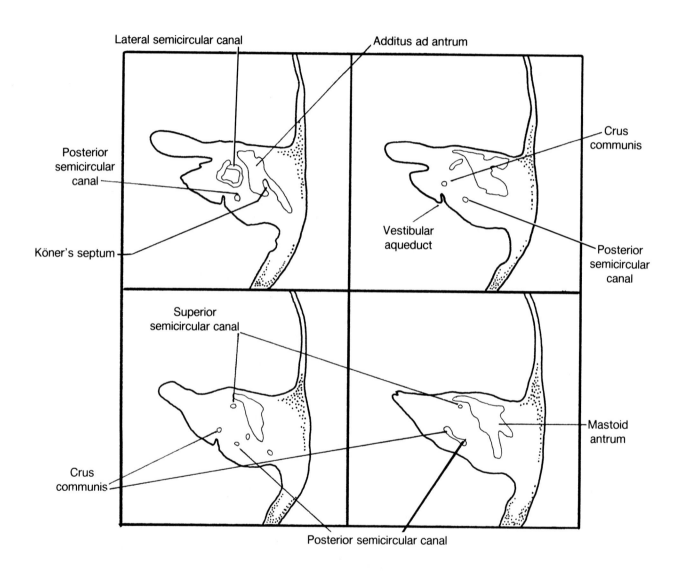

Lateral semicircular canal

Additus ad antrum

Posterior semicircular canal

Köner's septum

Crus communis

Vestibular aqueduct

Posterior semicircular canal

Superior semicircular canal

Crus communis

Mastoid antrum

Posterior semicircular canal

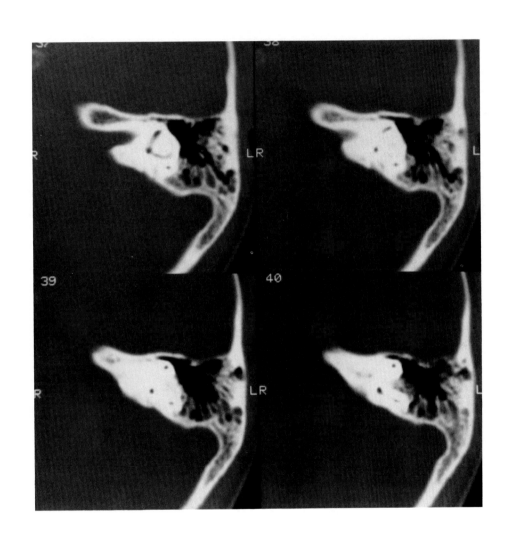

Superior semicircular canal

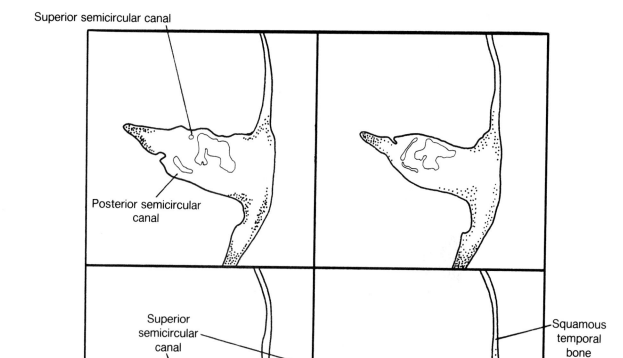

Posterior semicircular
canal

Superior
semicircular
canal

Squamous
temporal
bone

Mastoid
air cells

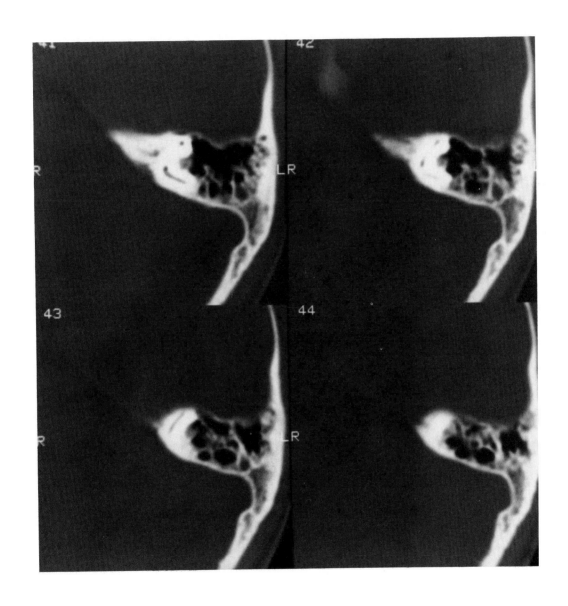

Temporal Bone: Coronal Plane

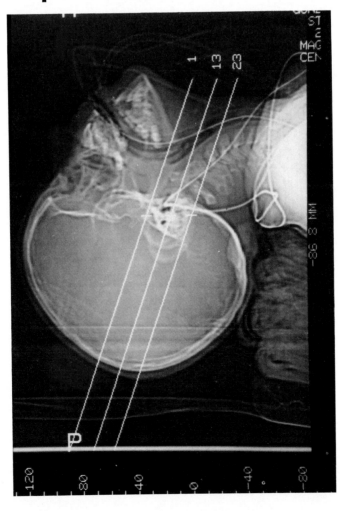

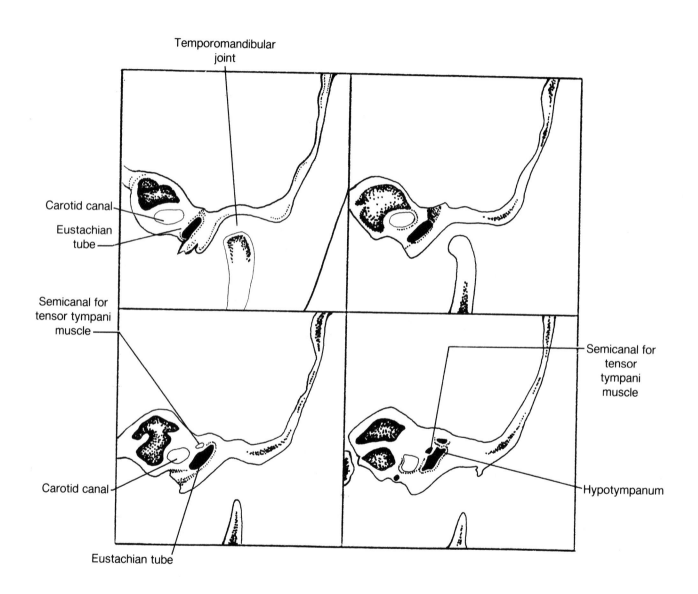

Temporomandibular
joint

Carotid canal

Eustachian
tube

Semicanal for
tensor tympani
muscle

Carotid canal

Eustachian tube

Semicanal for
tensor
tympani
muscle

Hypotympanum

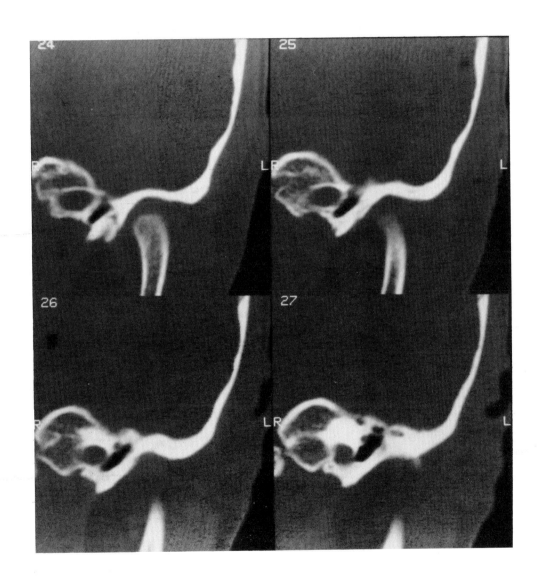

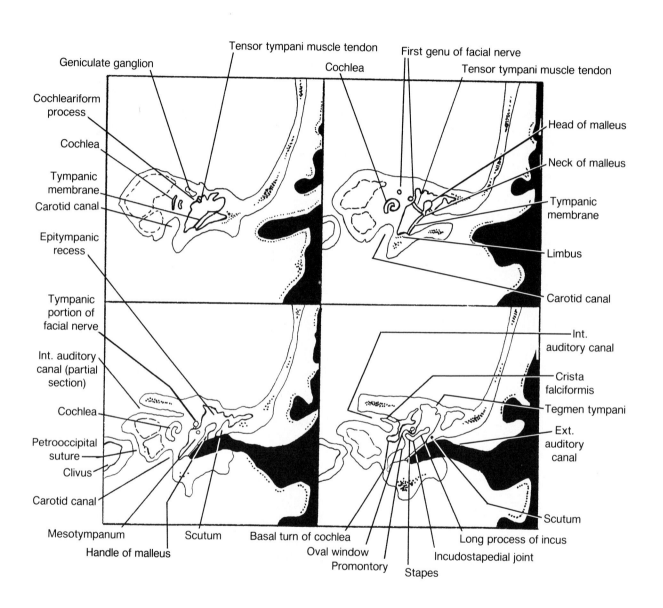

Geniculate ganglion

Tensor tympani muscle tendon

Cochlea

First genu of facial nerve

Tensor tympani muscle tendon

Cochleariform process

Head of malleus

Cochlea

Neck of malleus

Tympanic membrane

Carotid canal

Tympanic membrane

Epitympanic recess

Limbus

Tympanic portion of facial nerve

Carotid canal

Int. auditory canal (partial section)

Int. auditory canal

Crista falciformis

Cochlea

Tegmen tympani

Petrooccipital suture

Ext. auditory canal

Clivus

Carotid canal

Scutum

Mesotympanum

Scutum

Long process of incus

Handle of malleus

Basal turn of cochlea

Incudostapedial joint

Oval window

Promontory

Stapes

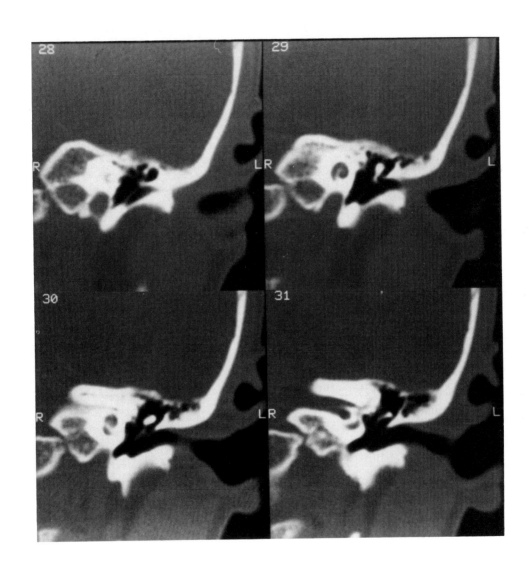

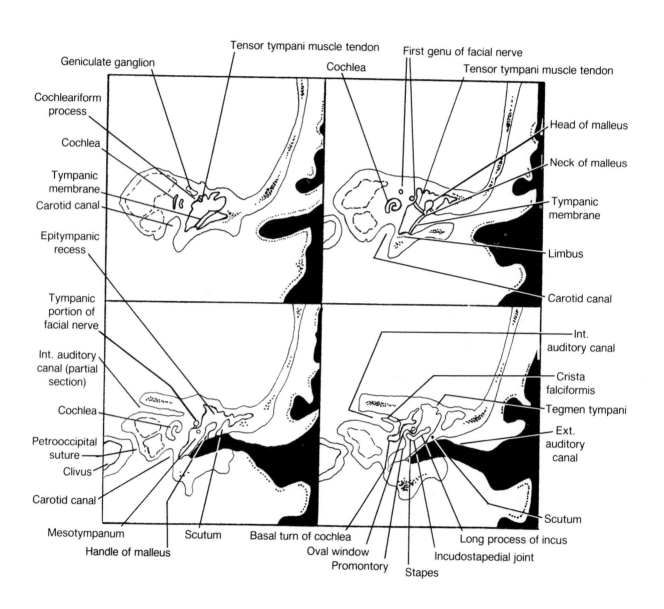

Geniculate ganglion

Tensor tympani muscle tendon

Cochlea

First genu of facial nerve

Tensor tympani muscle tendon

Cochleariform process

Cochlea

Tympanic membrane

Carotid canal

Epitympanic recess

Head of malleus

Neck of malleus

Tympanic membrane

Limbus

Carotid canal

Tympanic portion of facial nerve

Int. auditory canal (partial section)

Cochlea

Petrooccipital suture

Clivus

Carotid canal

Int. auditory canal

Crista falciformis

Tegmen tympani

Ext. auditory canal

Scutum

Mesotympanum

Handle of malleus

Scutum

Basal turn of cochlea

Oval window

Promontory

Stapes

Long process of incus

Incudostapedial joint

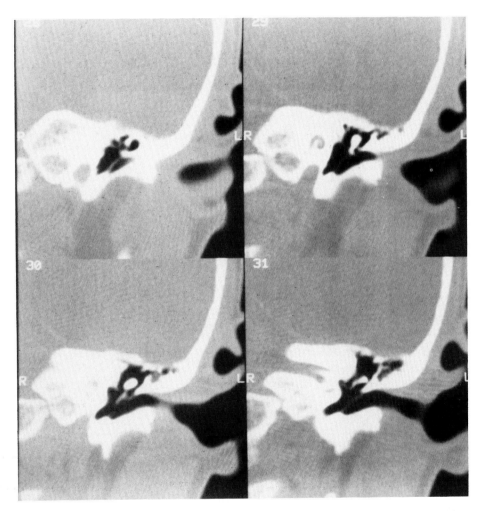

Images 28 through 31 are repeated from p 249 using a lighter photographic technique to emphasize fine detail in the middle ear.

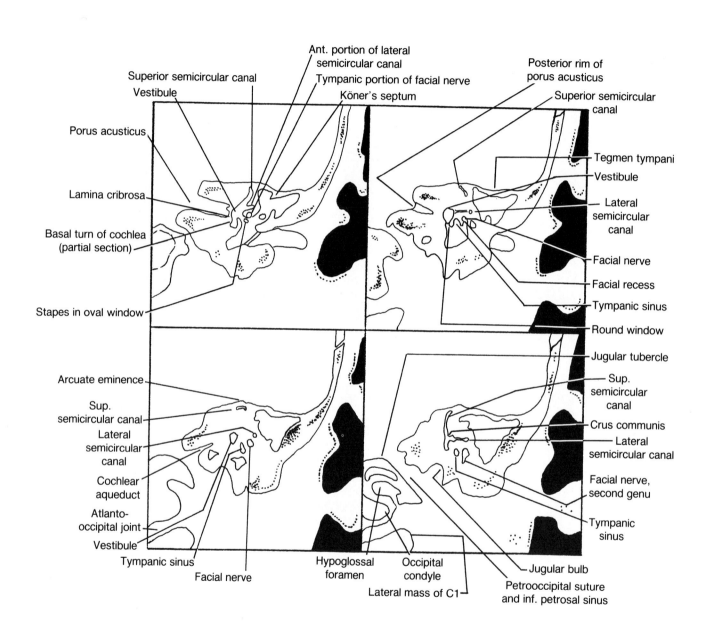

Ant. portion of lateral
semicircular canal

Tympanic portion of facial nerve

Köner's septum

Superior semicircular canal
Vestibule

Posterior rim of
porus acusticus

Superior semicircular
canal

Porus acusticus

Tegmen tympani

Vestibule

Lamina cribrosa

Lateral
semicircular
canal

Basal turn of cochlea
(partial section)

Facial nerve

Facial recess

Tympanic sinus

Stapes in oval window

Round window

Jugular tubercle

Arcuate eminence

Sup.
semicircular
canal

Sup.
semicircular canal

Crus communis

Lateral
semicircular
canal

Lateral
semicircular canal

Cochlear
aqueduct

Facial nerve,
second genu

Atlanto-
occipital joint

Tympanic
sinus

Vestibule

Tympanic sinus

Facial nerve

Hypoglossal
foramen

Occipital
condyle

Jugular bulb

Petrooccipital suture
and inf. petrosal sinus

Lateral mass of C1

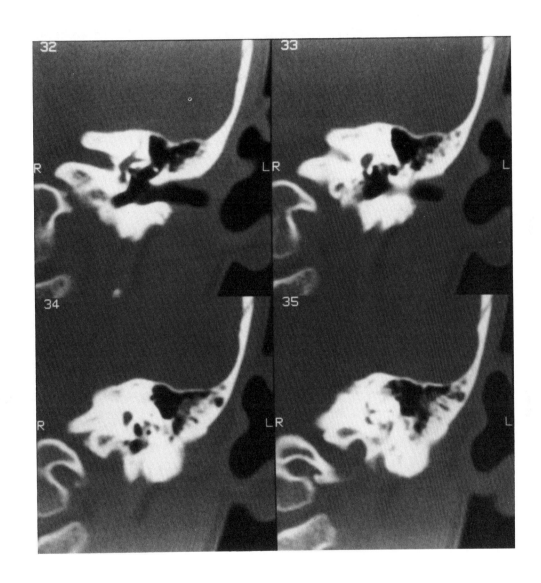

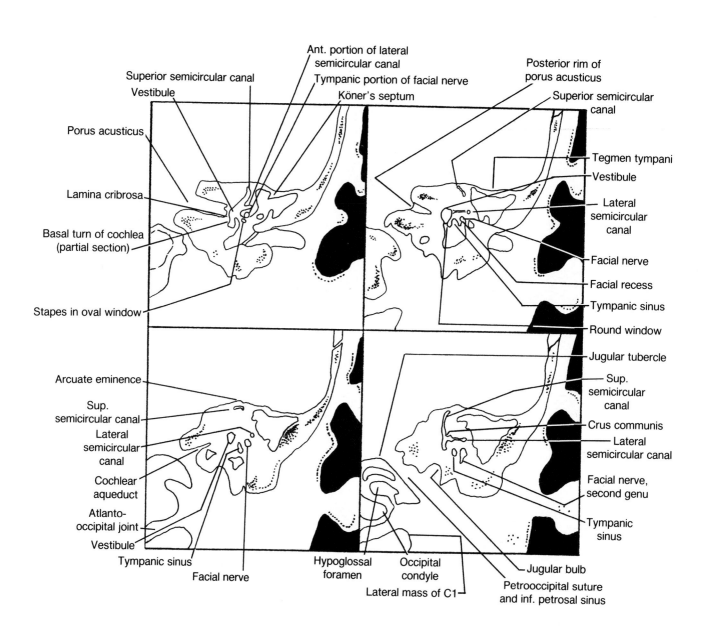

Ant. portion of lateral
semicircular canal

Superior semicircular canal
Vestibule

Tympanic portion of facial nerve

Köner's septum

Posterior rim of
porus acusticus

Superior semicircular
canal

Porus acusticus

Tegmen tympani

Vestibule

Lateral
semicircular
canal

Lamina cribrosa

Basal turn of cochlea
(partial section)

Facial nerve

Facial recess

Tympanic sinus

Stapes in oval window

Round window

Jugular tubercle

Arcuate eminence

Sup.
semicircular
canal

Crus communis

Sup.
semicircular canal

Lateral
semicircular
canal

Lateral
semicircular canal

Cochlear
aqueduct

Facial nerve,
second genu

Atlanto-
occipital joint

Tympanic
sinus

Vestibule

Tympanic sinus

Facial nerve

Hypoglossal
foramen

Occipital
condyle

Jugular bulb

Lateral mass of C1

Petrooccipital suture
and inf. petrosal sinus

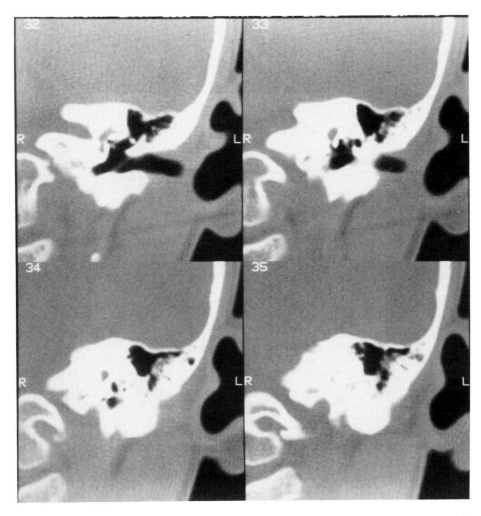

Images 32 through 35 are repeated from p 253 using a lighter photographic technique to emphasize fine detail in the middle ear.

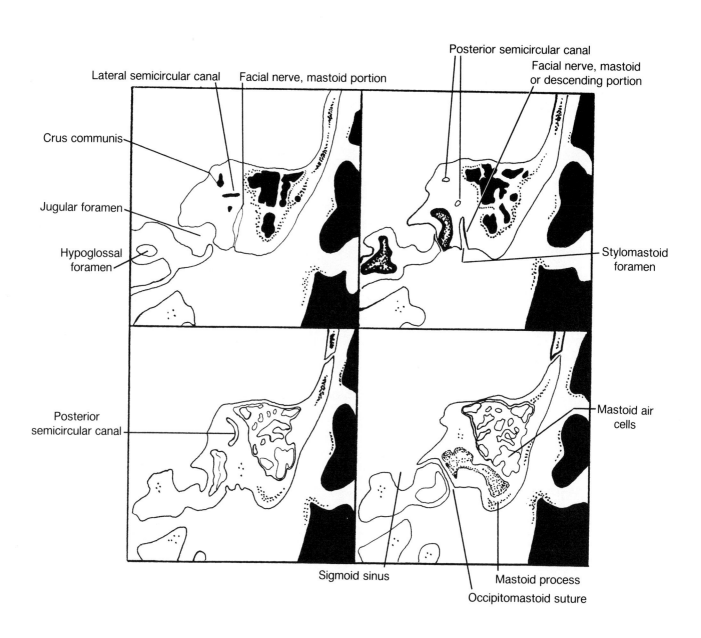

Lateral semicircular canal

Facial nerve, mastoid portion

Posterior semicircular canal

Facial nerve, mastoid or descending portion

Crus communis

Jugular foramen

Hypoglossal foramen

Stylomastoid foramen

Posterior semicircular canal

Mastoid air cells

Sigmoid sinus

Mastoid process

Occipitomastoid suture

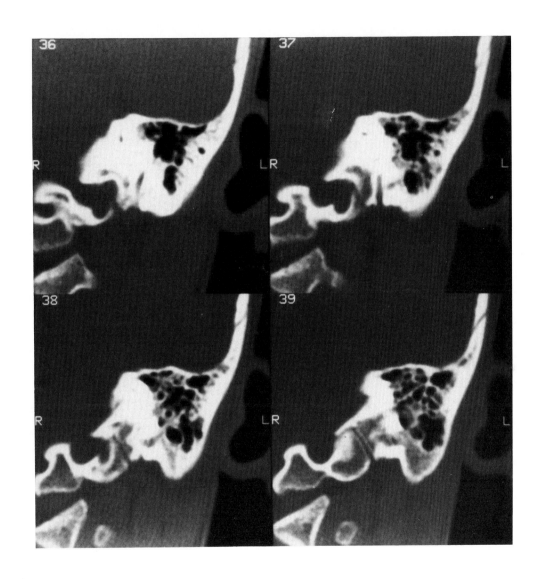

6 | Spine

UPPER CERVICAL SPINE
MID- AND LOWER CERVICAL SPINE
THORACIC SPINE
CONUS MEDULLARIS
LUMBAR SPINE

CERVICAL SPINE

Although the upper cervical spine and craniocervical junction offer better natural contrast than the mid- and lower cervical spine, intrathecal administration of water-soluble contrast medium prior to CT scanning is indicated when definition of neural structures is essential. In general, 3-mm contiguous sections at 3-mm intervals are used, with orientation through the disk spaces as much as possible. This protocol may be supplemented with 1.5-mm sections through individual disk spaces when necessary. Long sections of the cervical spine require 5-mm sections at 5-mm intervals, but this will decrease the quality of reformatted images.

THORACIC SPINE

In the thoracic spine, axial scans without intrathecal contrast delineate the bony structures, including fractures and their relation to the bony spinal canal. However, delineation of the cord requires intrathecal contrast. Contiguous 3-mm sections are selected for reformatting of short segments (three or four vertebral bodies), and 5-mm sections at 5-mm intervals for longer segments of the spine.

LUMBAR SPINE

Evaluation of the lumbosacral spine for disk disease requires 3-mm sections at 3-mm intervals angled through the disk spaces. In larger patients, 5-mm sections at 3-mm intervals may be preferred. The scan extends from pedicle to pedicle at each level. Reformatted images are quite helpful if motion has not been a problem.

Postoperatively, CT scans following the intrathecal administration of contrast medium are recommended. Contiguous sections may be necessary when evaluating areas of previous surgical fusion or in cases of spinal stenosis. Scans are performed approximately 4 hours following myelography. The patient should be rotated 360° immediately prior to scanning in order to prevent layering of the contrast medium. Scans with the patient in the prone position may occasionally be necessary to define the anterior limit of the thecal sac when layering does occur. Scans may be performed immediately after administering low dose intrathecal contrast without myelography.

The reformatted coronal images of the noncontrast scan at the L5–S1 level illustrated in this chapter show asymmetries of the nerve roots, which may be visible because of slight patient tilt that, in this instance, should not be interpreted as pathologic asymmetry. A more symmetrical coronal reformat is provided with the contrast CT of the L5–S1 region.

Upper Cervical Spine without Intrathecal Contrast

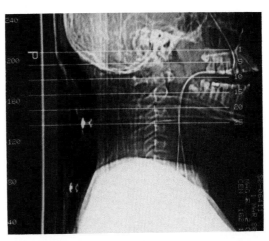

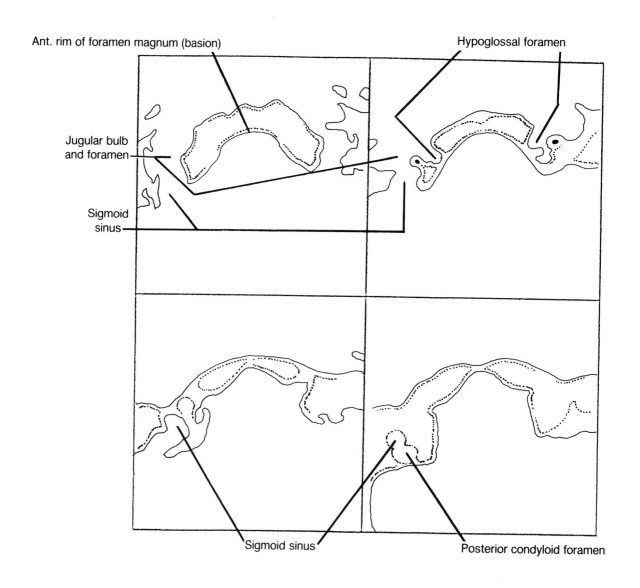

Ant. rim of foramen magnum (basion)

Hypoglossal foramen

Jugular bulb
and foramen

Sigmoid
sinus

Sigmoid sinus

Posterior condyloid foramen

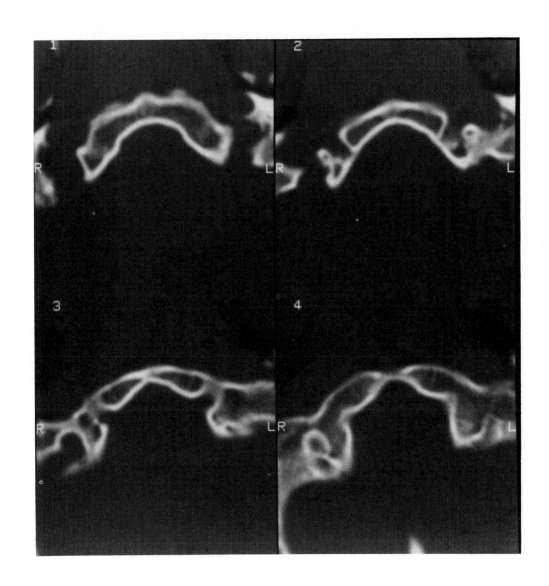

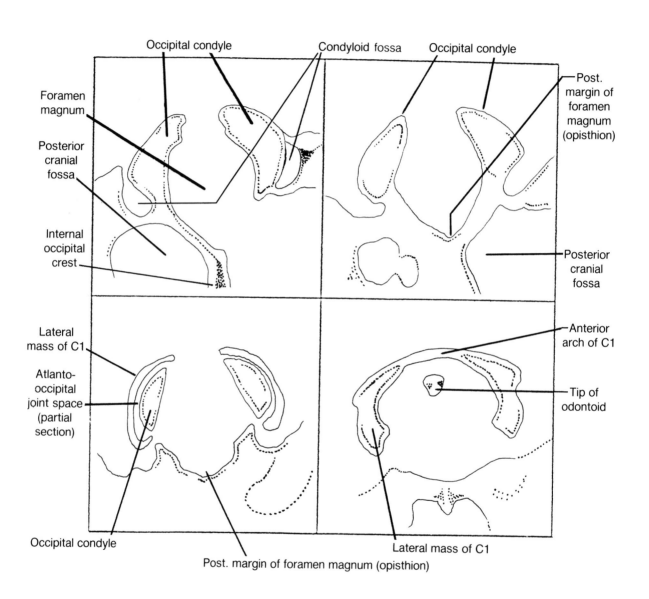

Occipital condyle

Condyloid fossa

Occipital condyle

Foramen magnum

Posterior cranial fossa

Internal occipital crest

Post. margin of foramen magnum (opisthion)

Posterior cranial fossa

Lateral mass of C1

Atlanto-occipital joint space (partial section)

Anterior arch of C1

Tip of odontoid

Occipital condyle

Post. margin of foramen magnum (opisthion)

Lateral mass of C1

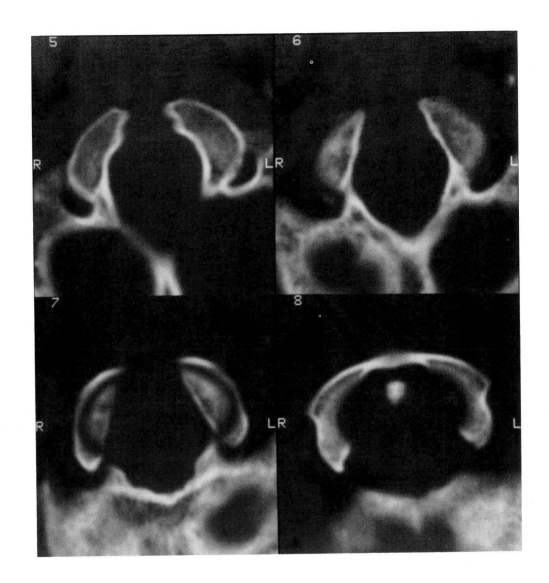

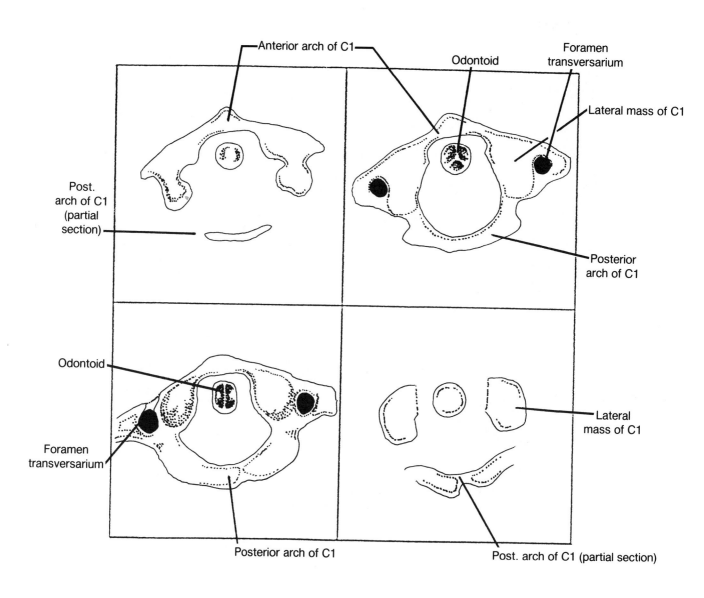

Anterior arch of C1

Odontoid

Foramen transversarium

Lateral mass of C1

Post. arch of C1 (partial section)

Posterior arch of C1

Odontoid

Foramen transversarium

Posterior arch of C1

Lateral mass of C1

Post. arch of C1 (partial section)

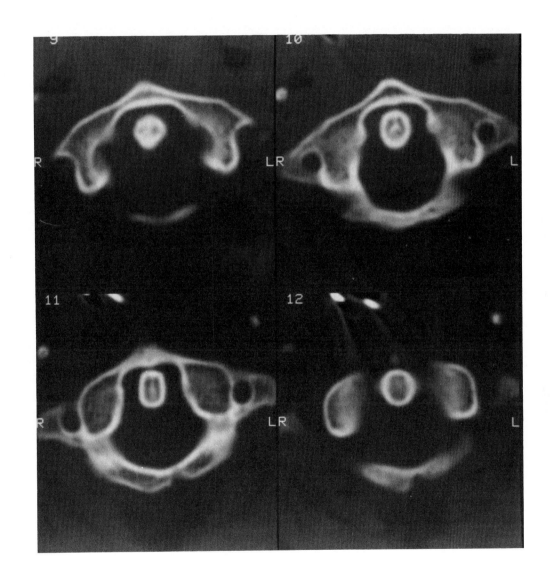

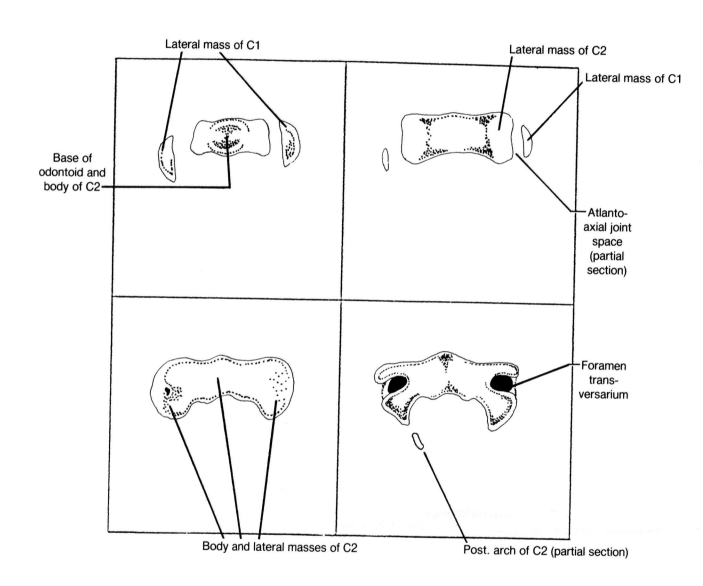

Lateral mass of C1

Lateral mass of C2

Lateral mass of C1

Base of odontoid and body of C2

Atlanto-axial joint space (partial section)

Foramen trans-versarium

Body and lateral masses of C2

Post. arch of C2 (partial section)

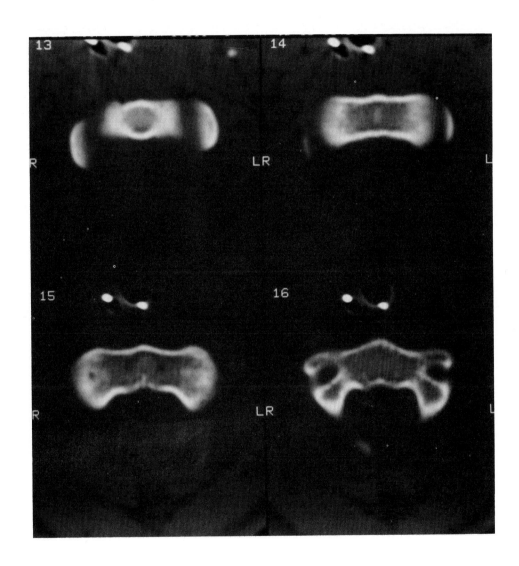

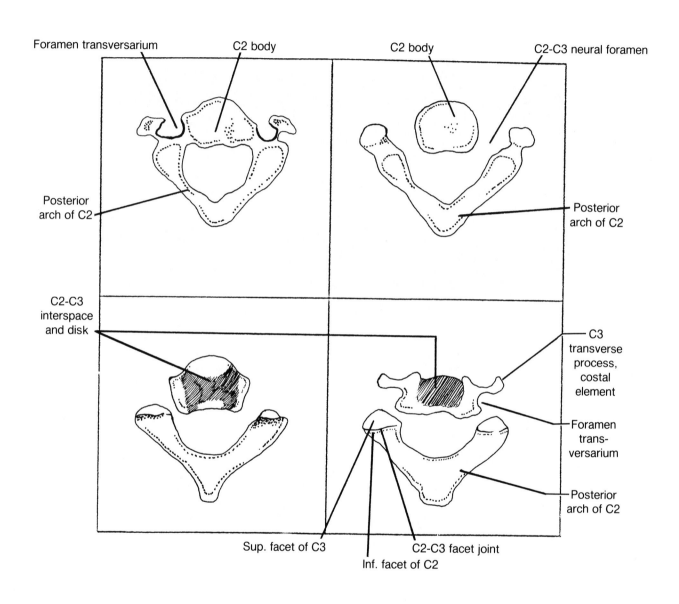

Foramen transversarium   C2 body

C2 body   C2-C3 neural foramen

Posterior arch of C2

Posterior arch of C2

C2-C3 interspace and disk

C3 transverse process, costal element

Foramen transversarium

Posterior arch of C2

Sup. facet of C3

Inf. facet of C2

C2-C3 facet joint

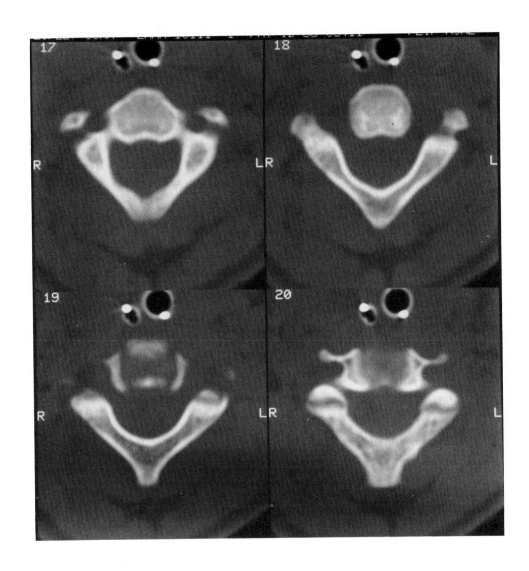

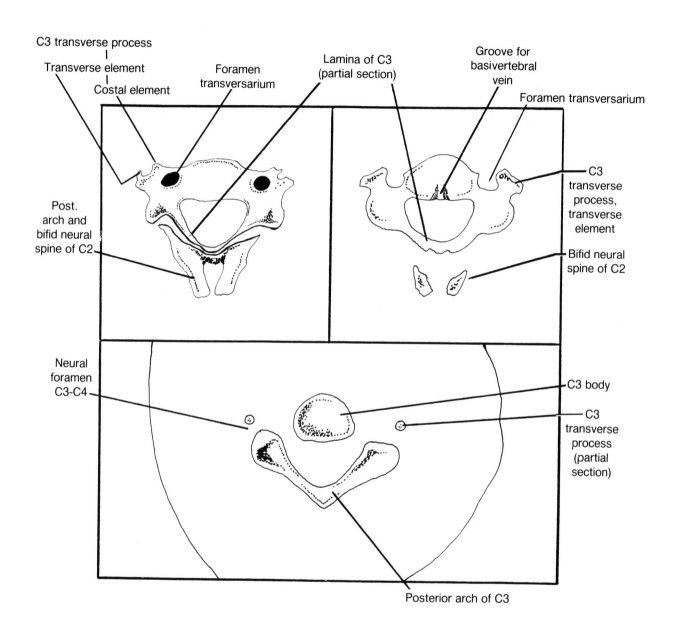

C3 transverse process

Transverse element

Costal element

Foramen transversarium

Lamina of C3 (partial section)

Groove for basivertebral vein

Foramen transversarium

C3 transverse process, transverse element

Post. arch and bifid neural spine of C2

Bifid neural spine of C2

Neural foramen C3-C4

C3 body

C3 transverse process (partial section)

Posterior arch of C3

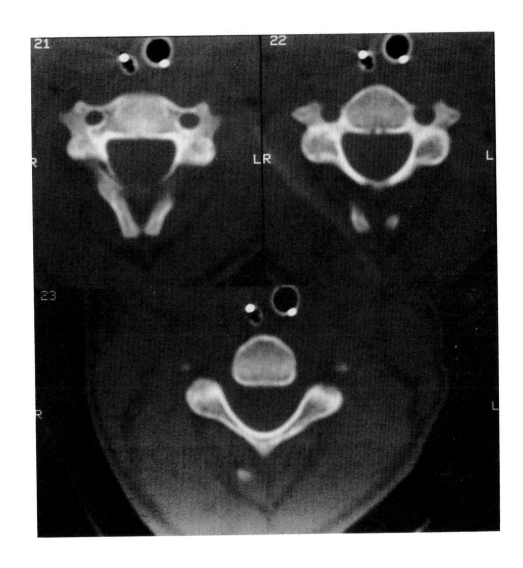

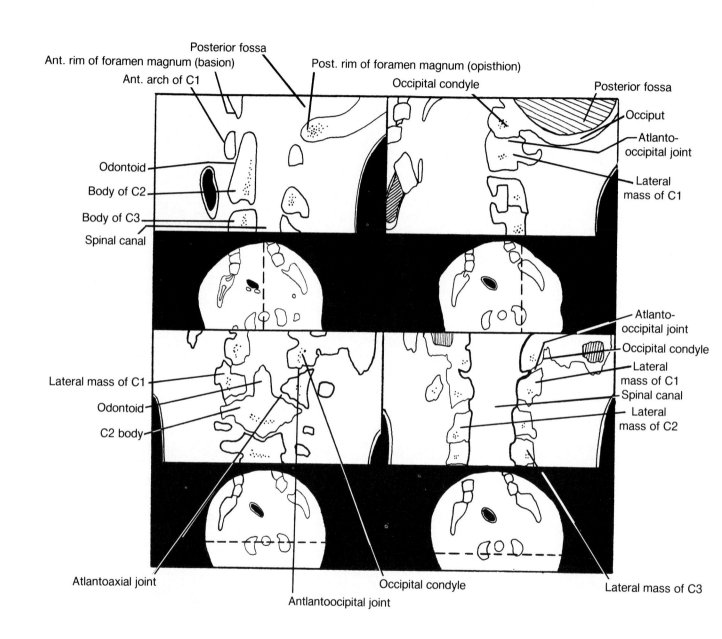

Posterior fossa

Ant. rim of foramen magnum (basion)
Ant. arch of C1

Post. rim of foramen magnum (opisthion)

Occipital condyle

Posterior fossa

Occiput

Atlanto-
occipital joint

Odontoid

Lateral
mass of C1

Body of C2

Body of C3

Spinal canal

Atlanto-
occipital joint

Occipital condyle

Lateral mass of C1

Lateral
mass of C1

Odontoid

Spinal canal

C2 body

Lateral
mass of C2

Atlantoaxial joint

Occipital condyle

Lateral mass of C3

Antlantoocipital joint

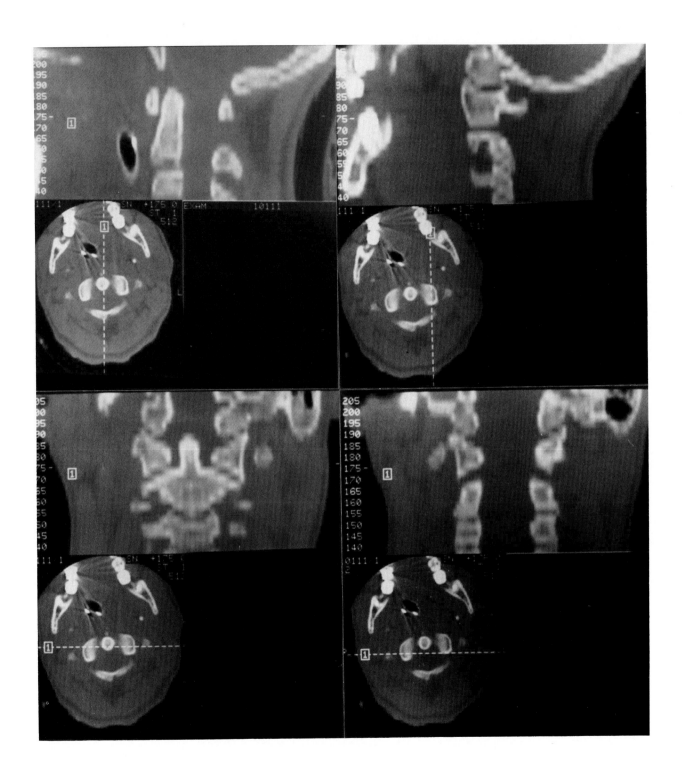

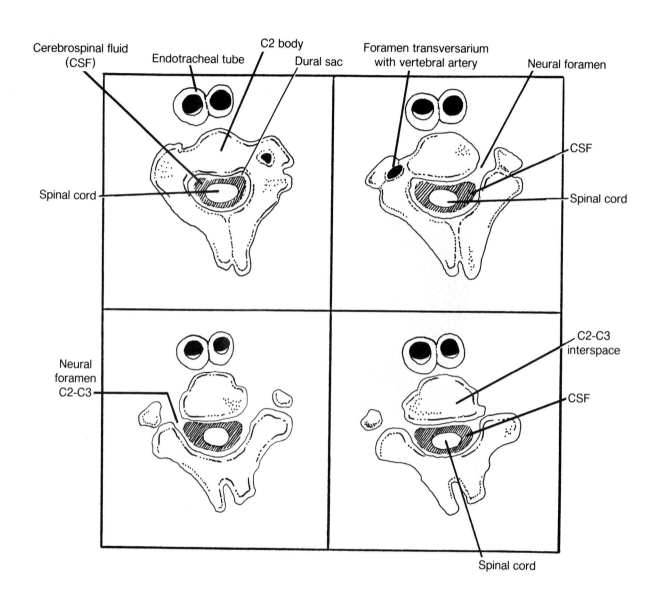

Cerebrospinal fluid (CSF)

Endotracheal tube

C2 body

Dural sac

Foramen transversarium with vertebral artery

Neural foramen

Spinal cord

CSF

Spinal cord

Neural foramen C2-C3

C2-C3 interspace

CSF

Spinal cord

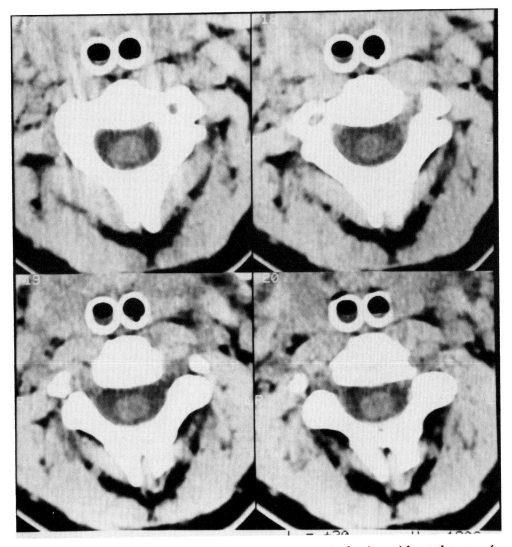

The spinal cord can usually be seen in the upper cervical spine without the use of intrathecal contrast.

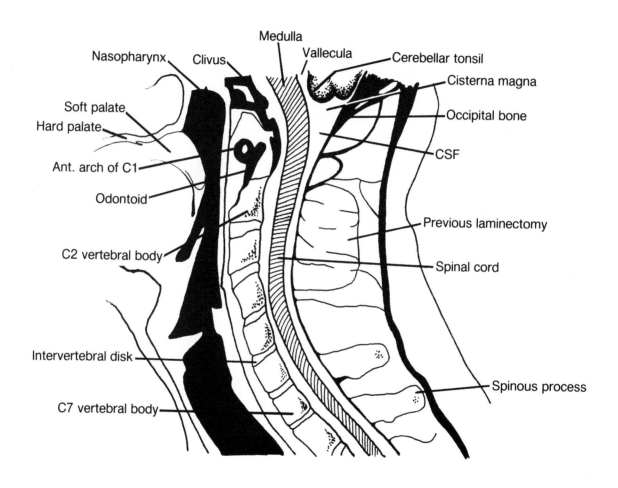

Nasopharynx

Clivus

Medulla

Vallecula

Cerebellar tonsil

Cisterna magna

Soft palate

Hard palate

Occipital bone

Ant. arch of C1

CSF

Odontoid

C2 vertebral body

Previous laminectomy

Spinal cord

Intervertebral disk

C7 vertebral body

Spinous process

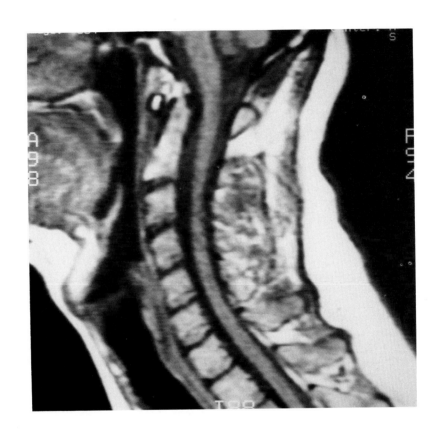

Mid- and Lower Cervical Spine with Intrathecal Contrast

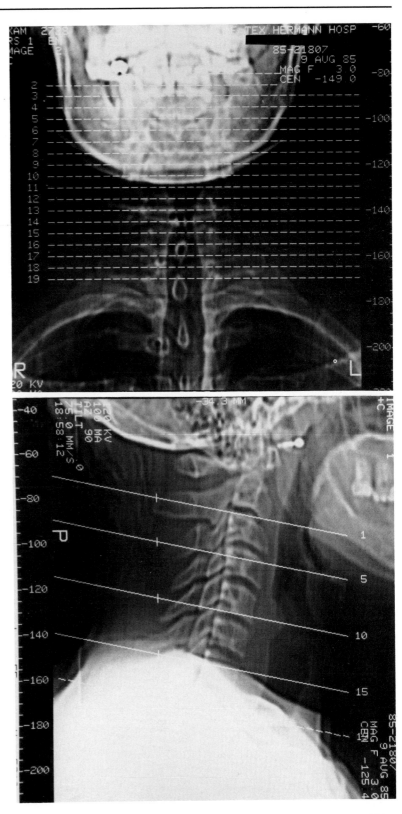

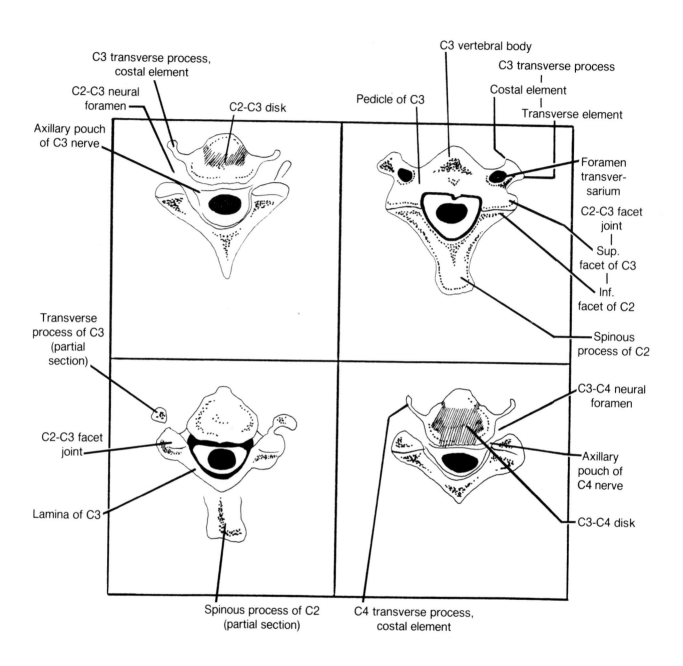

C3 transverse process, costal element

C3 vertebral body

C2-C3 neural foramen

C3 transverse process

Costal element

Axillary pouch of C3 nerve

Pedicle of C3

Transverse element

C2-C3 disk

Foramen transversarium

C2-C3 facet joint

Sup. facet of C3

Inf. facet of C2

Spinous process of C2

Transverse process of C3 (partial section)

C3-C4 neural foramen

C2-C3 facet joint

Axillary pouch of C4 nerve

Lamina of C3

C3-C4 disk

Spinous process of C2 (partial section)

C4 transverse process, costal element

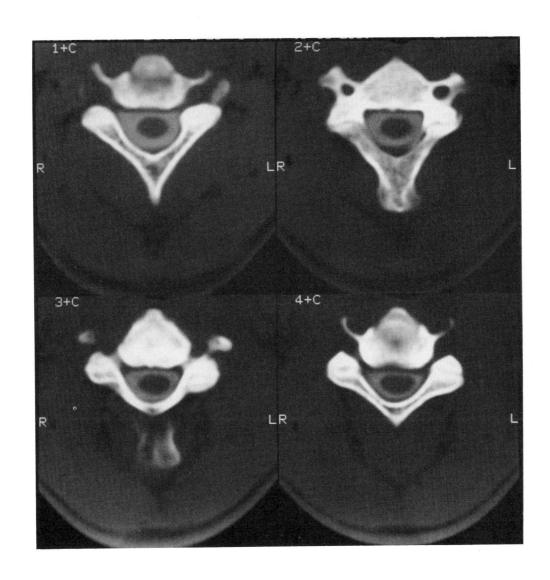

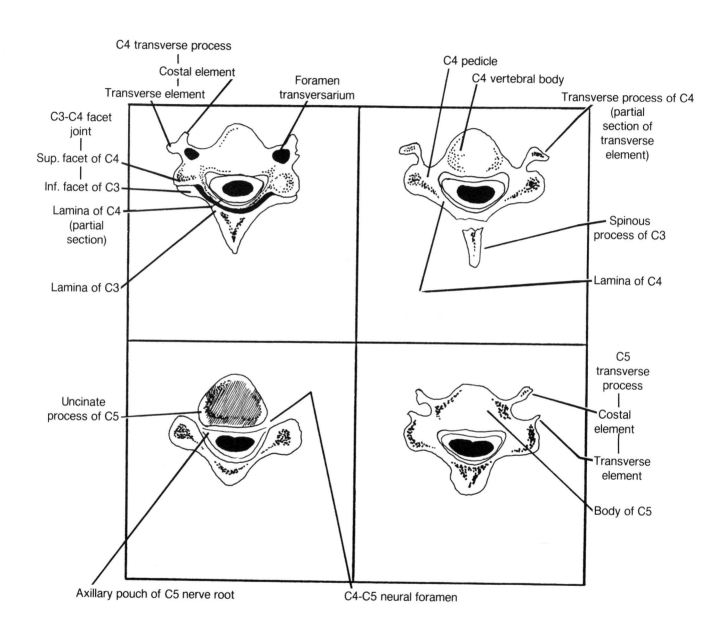

C4 transverse process
Costal element
Transverse element
Foramen transversarium

C3-C4 facet joint
Sup. facet of C4
Inf. facet of C3
Lamina of C4 (partial section)
Lamina of C3

C4 pedicle
C4 vertebral body
Transverse process of C4 (partial section of transverse element)
Spinous process of C3
Lamina of C4

Uncinate process of C5

C5 transverse process
Costal element
Transverse element
Body of C5

Axillary pouch of C5 nerve root

C4-C5 neural foramen

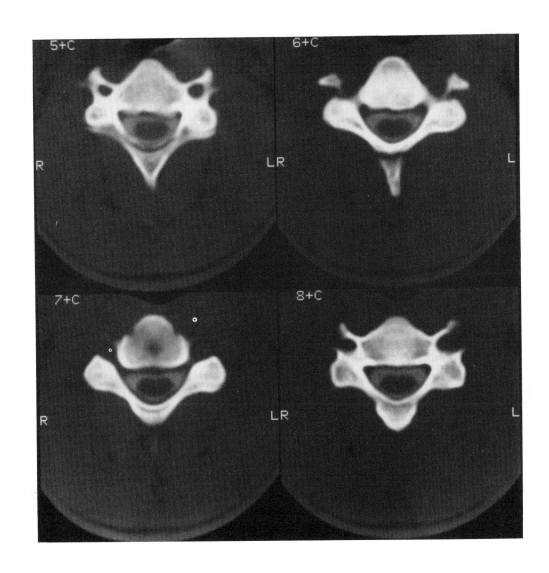

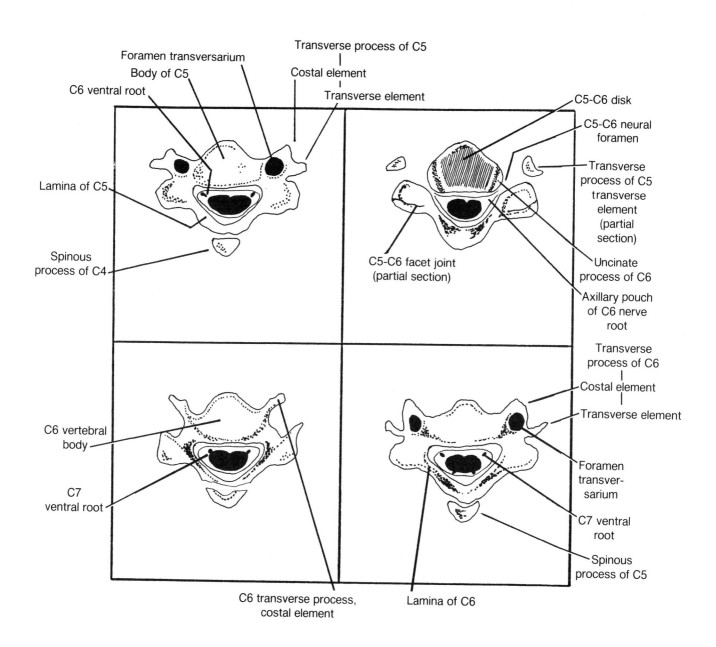

Foramen transversarium
Body of C5
C6 ventral root
Transverse process of C5
Costal element
Transverse element

C5-C6 disk
C5-C6 neural foramen
Transverse process of C5 transverse element (partial section)

Lamina of C5
Spinous process of C4

C5-C6 facet joint (partial section)

Uncinate process of C6
Axillary pouch of C6 nerve root

Transverse process of C6
Costal element
Transverse element

C6 vertebral body
C7 ventral root

Foramen transversarium
C7 ventral root
Spinous process of C5

C6 transverse process, costal element

Lamina of C6

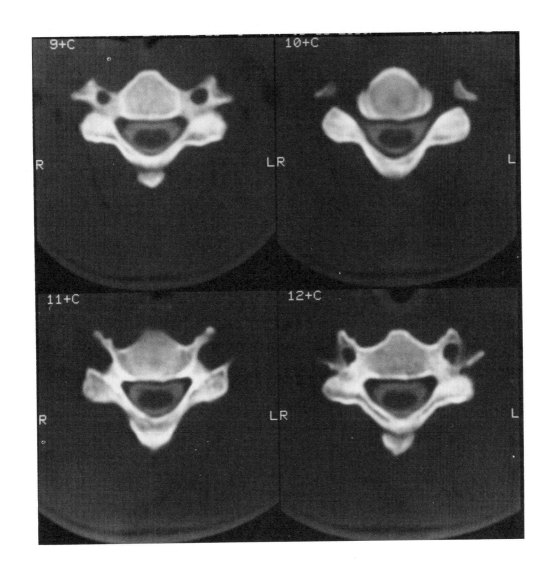

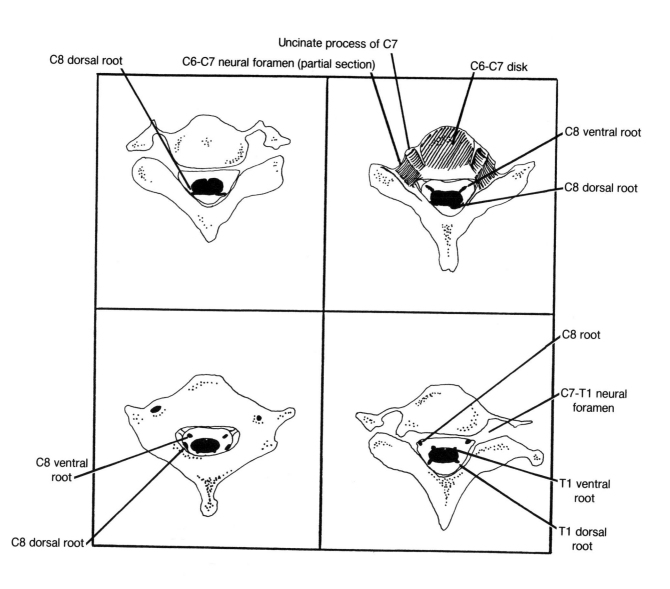

C8 dorsal root

C6-C7 neural foramen (partial section)

Uncinate process of C7

C6-C7 disk

C8 ventral root

C8 dorsal root

C8 ventral root

C8 dorsal root

C8 root

C7-T1 neural foramen

T1 ventral root

T1 dorsal root

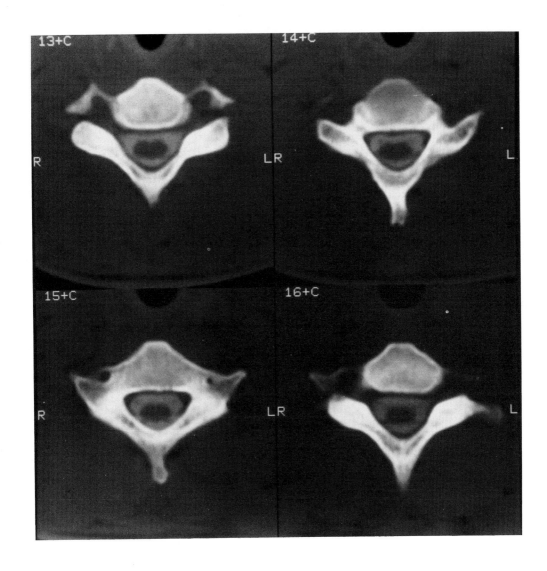

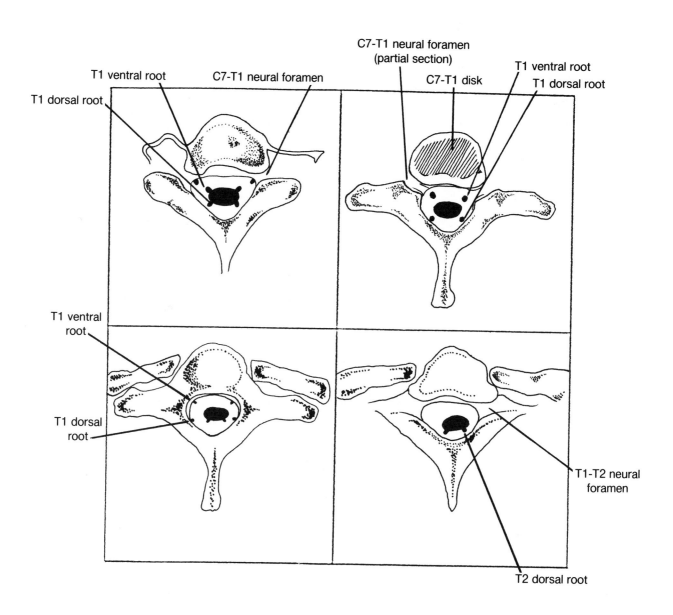

T1 dorsal root

T1 ventral root   C7-T1 neural foramen

C7-T1 neural foramen
(partial section)

C7-T1 disk   T1 ventral root
T1 dorsal root

T1 ventral
root

T1 dorsal
root

T1-T2 neural
foramen

T2 dorsal root

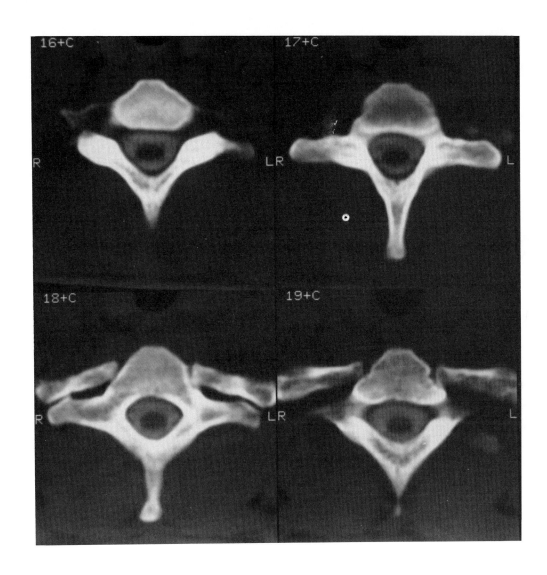

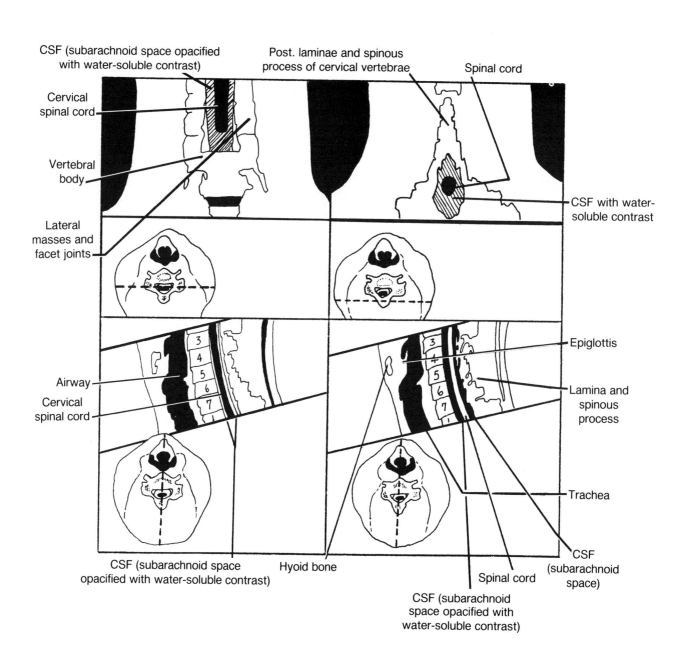

CSF (subarachnoid space opacified with water-soluble contrast)

Cervical spinal cord

Vertebral body

Lateral masses and facet joints

Post. laminae and spinous process of cervical vertebrae

Spinal cord

CSF with water-soluble contrast

Airway

Cervical spinal cord

Epiglottis

Lamina and spinous process

Trachea

CSF (subarachnoid space)

CSF (subarachnoid space opacified with water-soluble contrast)

Hyoid bone

Spinal cord

CSF (subarachnoid space opacified with water-soluble contrast)

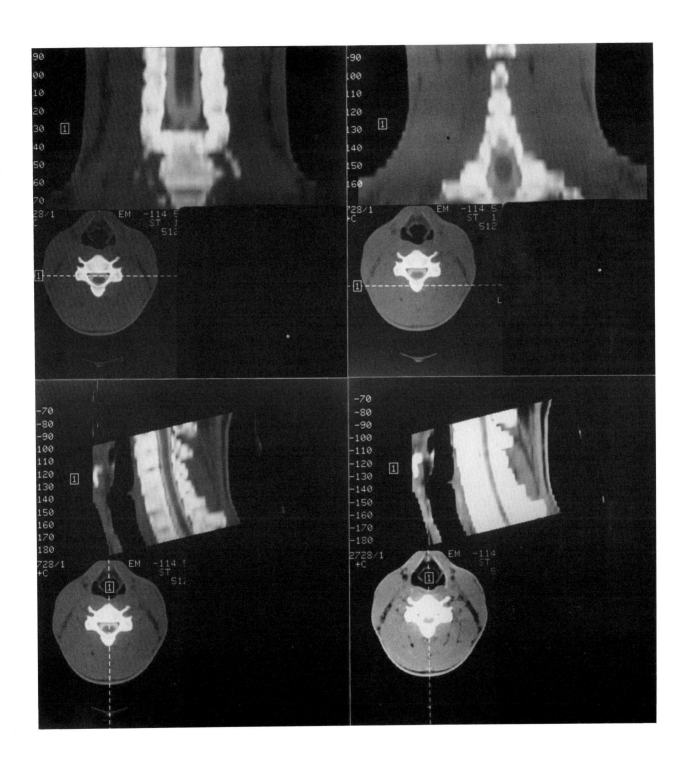

Midcervical Spine without Intrathecal Contrast

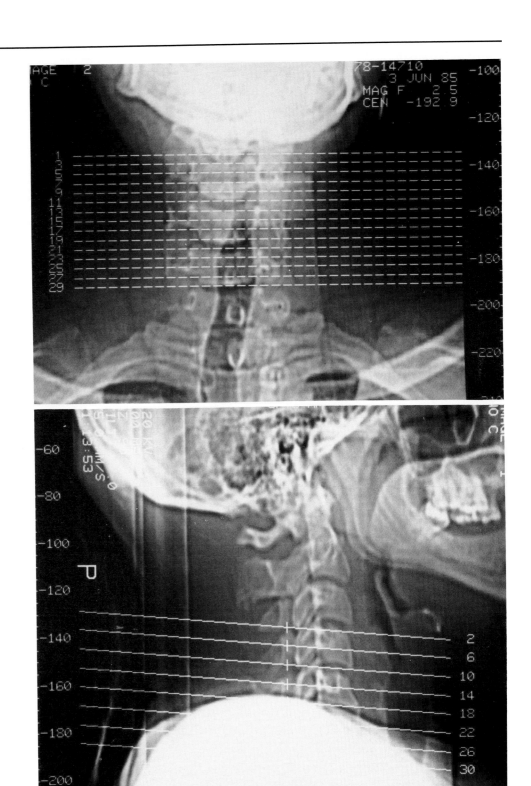

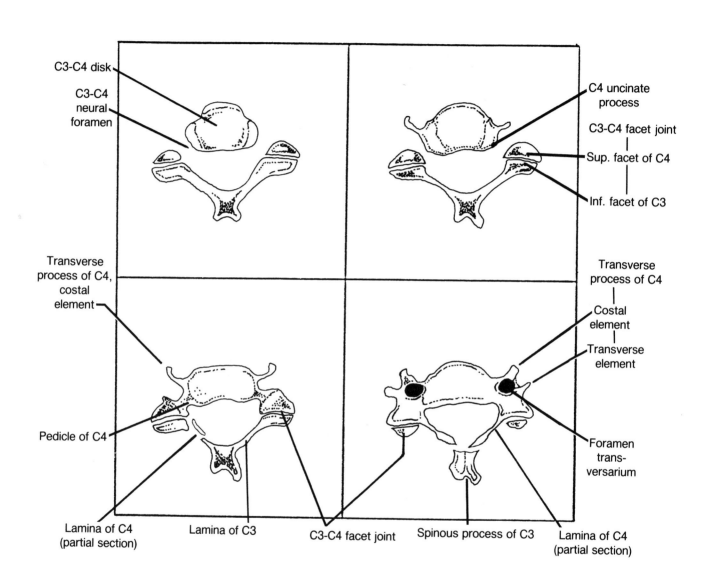

C3-C4 disk

C3-C4 neural foramen

C4 uncinate process

C3-C4 facet joint

Sup. facet of C4

Inf. facet of C3

Transverse process of C4, costal element

Transverse process of C4

Costal element

Transverse element

Pedicle of C4

Foramen trans-versarium

Lamina of C4 (partial section)

Lamina of C3

C3-C4 facet joint

Spinous process of C3

Lamina of C4 (partial section)

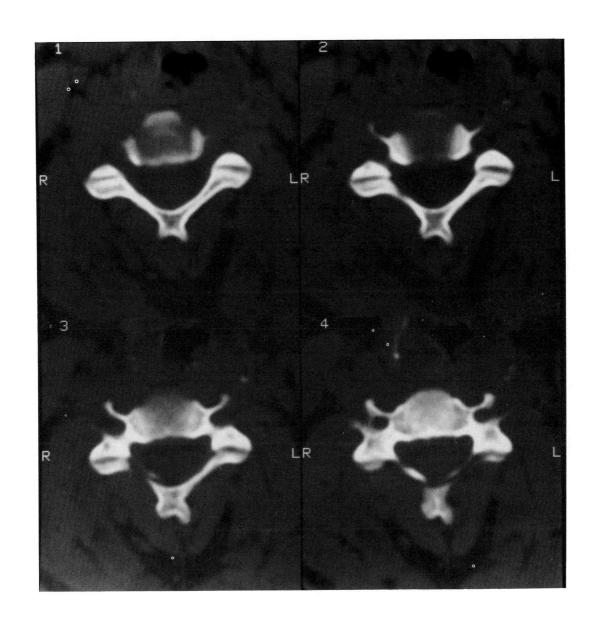

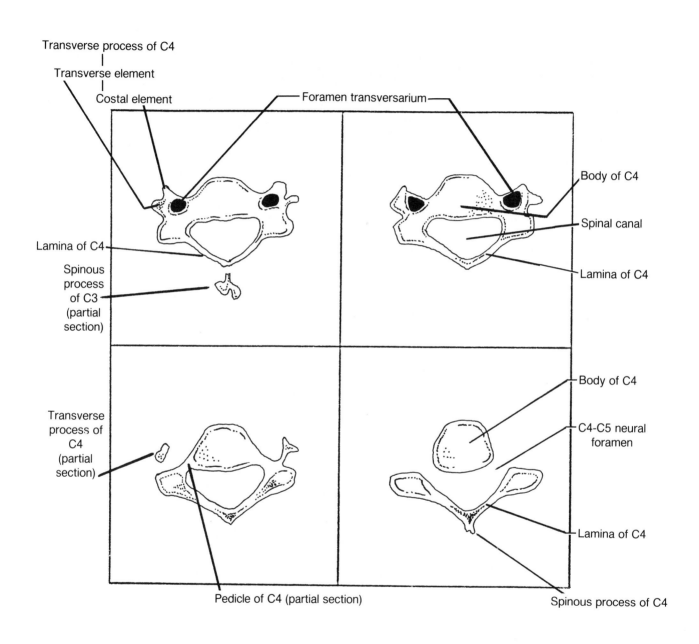

Transverse process of C4

Transverse element

Costal element

Foramen transversarium

Body of C4

Spinal canal

Lamina of C4

Lamina of C4

Spinous process of C3 (partial section)

Transverse process of C4 (partial section)

Body of C4

C4-C5 neural foramen

Lamina of C4

Spinous process of C4

Pedicle of C4 (partial section)

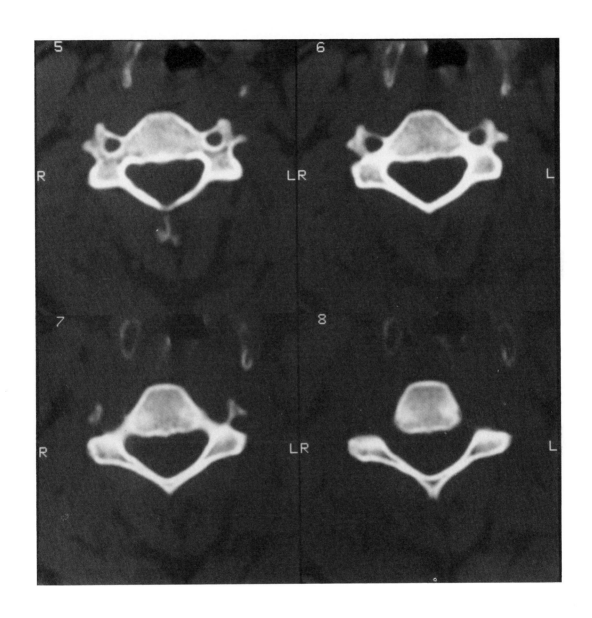

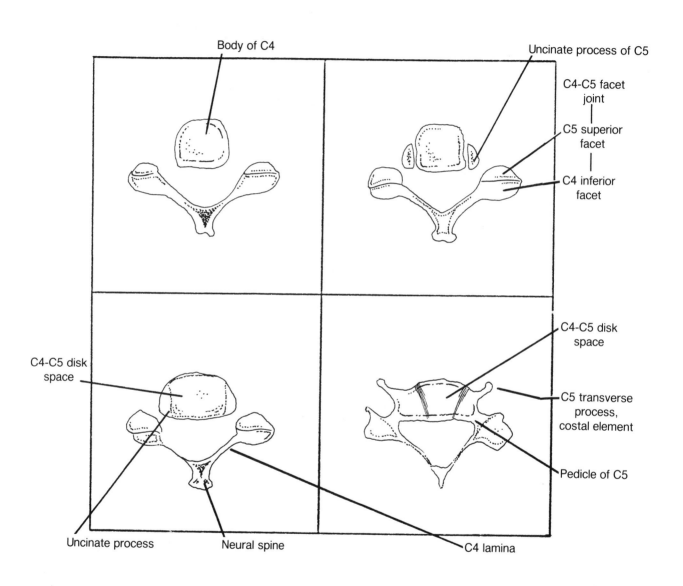

Body of C4

Uncinate process of C5

C4-C5 facet joint

C5 superior facet

C4 inferior facet

C4-C5 disk space

C4-C5 disk space

C5 transverse process, costal element

Pedicle of C5

Uncinate process

Neural spine

C4 lamina

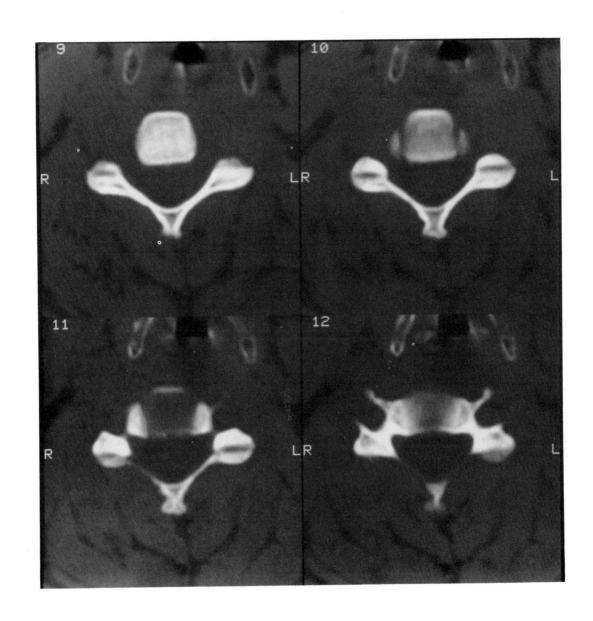

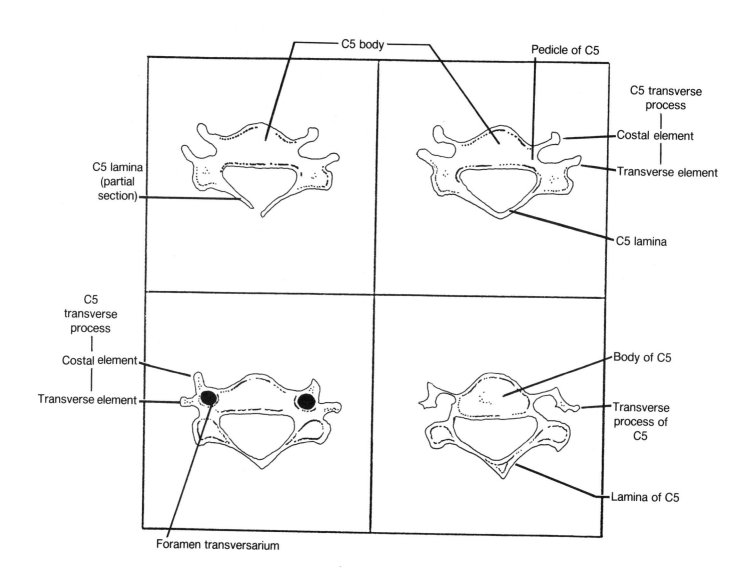

C5 body — Pedicle of C5

C5 transverse process
Costal element
Transverse element

C5 lamina (partial section)

C5 lamina

C5 transverse process
Costal element
Transverse element

Body of C5

Transverse process of C5

Lamina of C5

Foramen transversarium

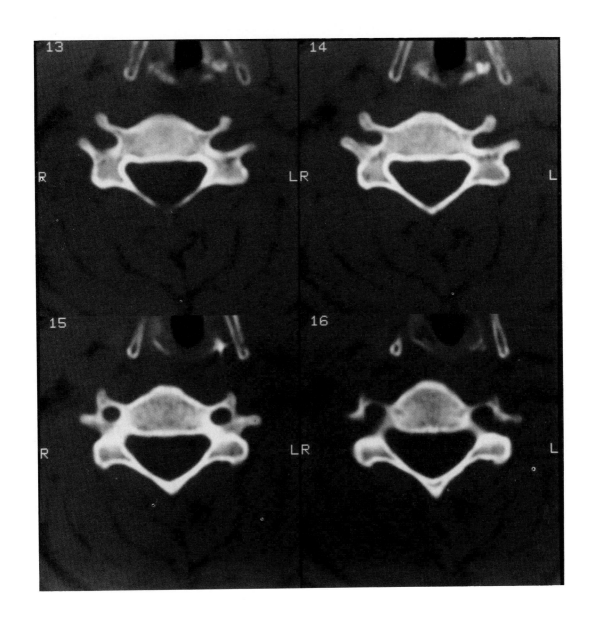

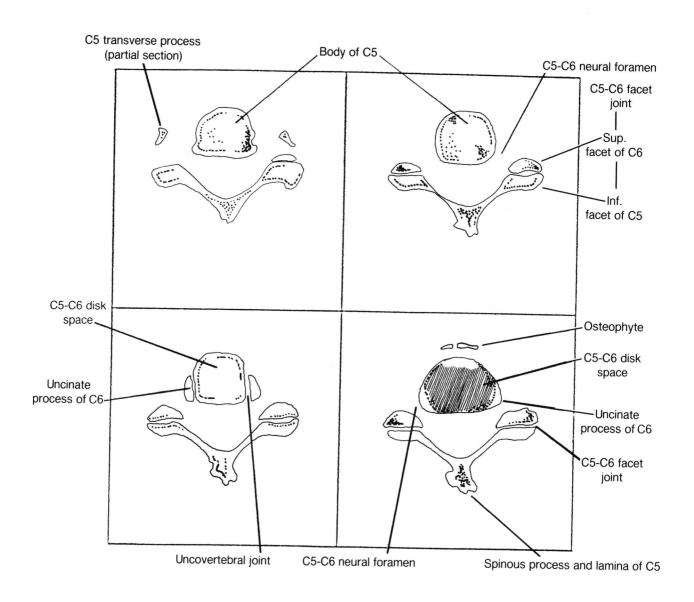

C5 transverse process (partial section)

Body of C5

C5-C6 neural foramen

C5-C6 facet joint

Sup. facet of C6

Inf. facet of C5

C5-C6 disk space

Osteophyte

C5-C6 disk space

Uncinate process of C6

Uncinate process of C6

C5-C6 facet joint

Uncovertebral joint

C5-C6 neural foramen

Spinous process and lamina of C5

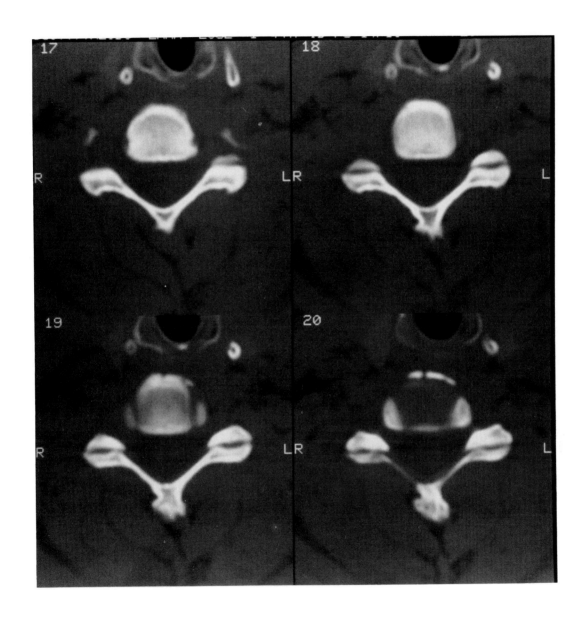

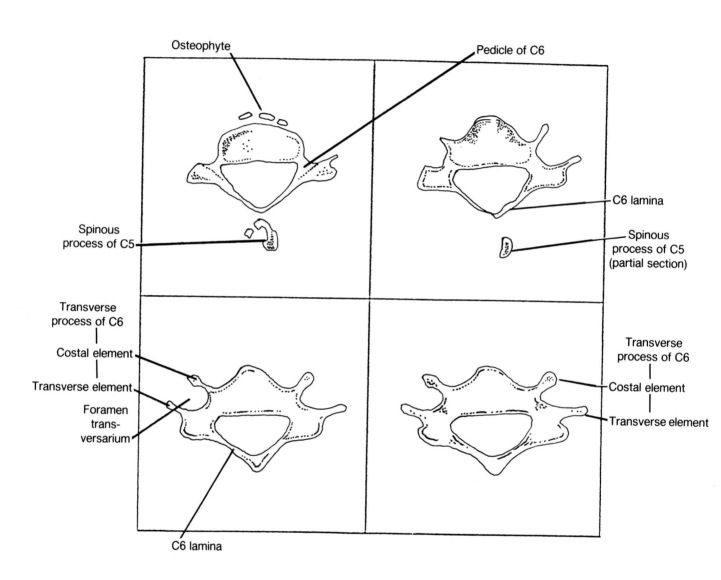

Osteophyte

Pedicle of C6

C6 lamina

Spinous process of C5

Spinous process of C5 (partial section)

Transverse process of C6

Costal element

Transverse element

Foramen transversarium

Transverse process of C6

Costal element

Transverse element

C6 lamina

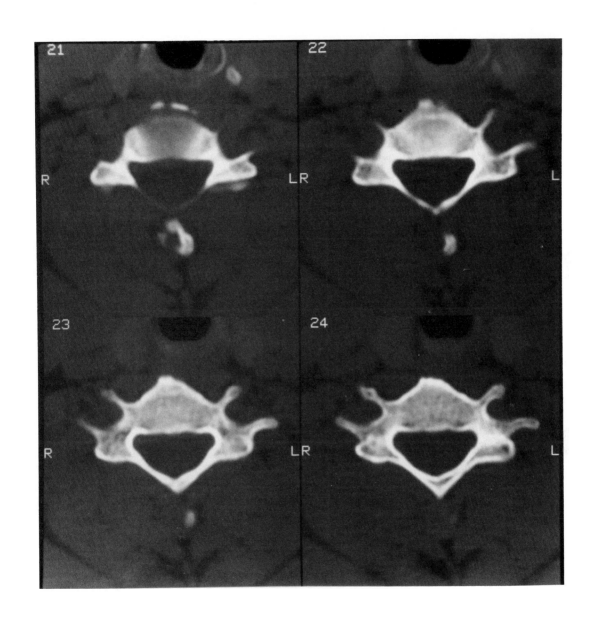

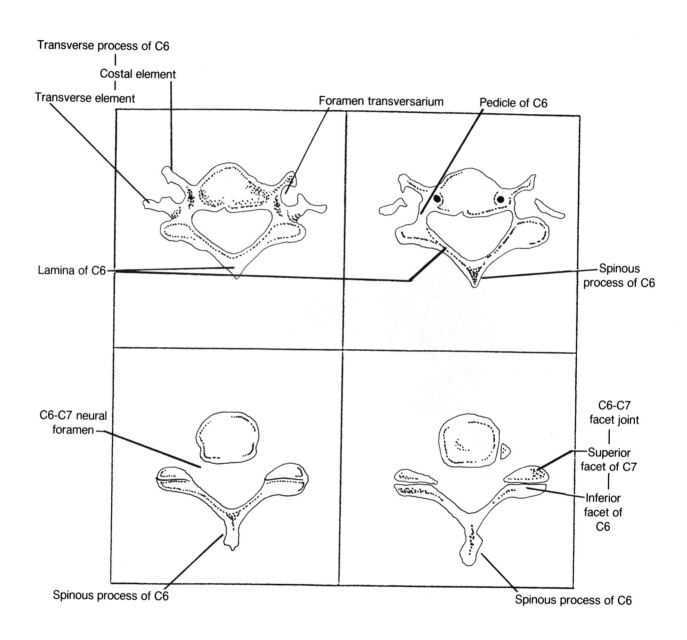

Transverse process of C6

Costal element

Transverse element

Foramen transversarium

Pedicle of C6

Lamina of C6

Spinous process of C6

C6-C7 neural foramen

C6-C7 facet joint

Superior facet of C7

Inferior facet of C6

Spinous process of C6

Spinous process of C6

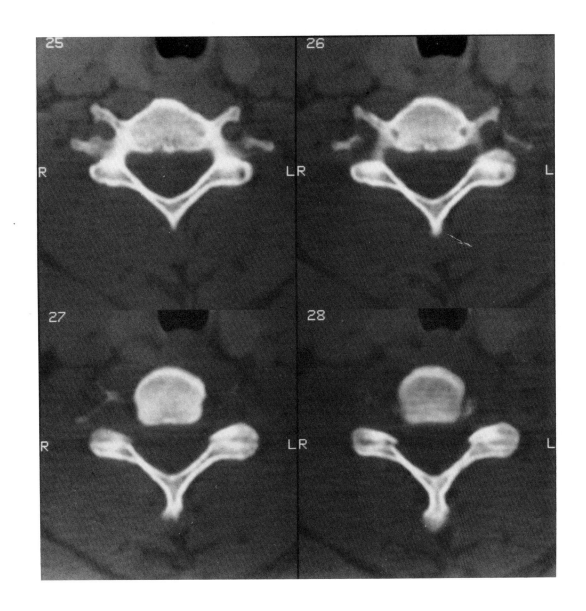

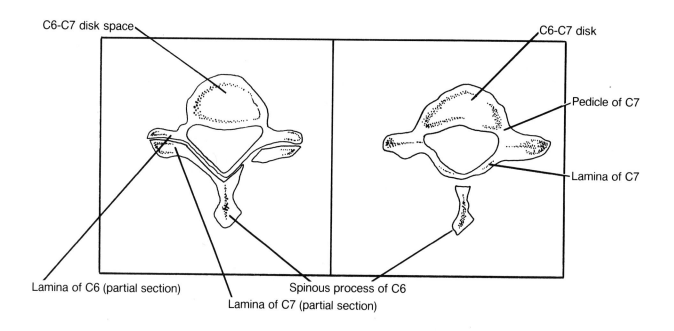

C6-C7 disk space

C6-C7 disk

Pedicle of C7

Lamina of C7

Lamina of C6 (partial section)

Spinous process of C6

Lamina of C7 (partial section)

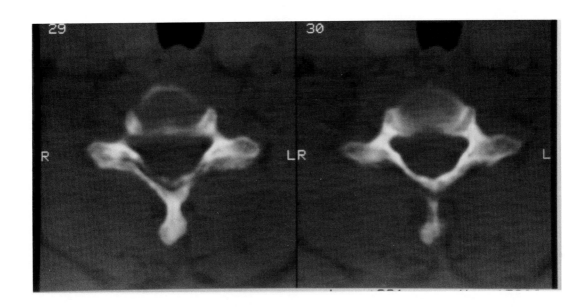

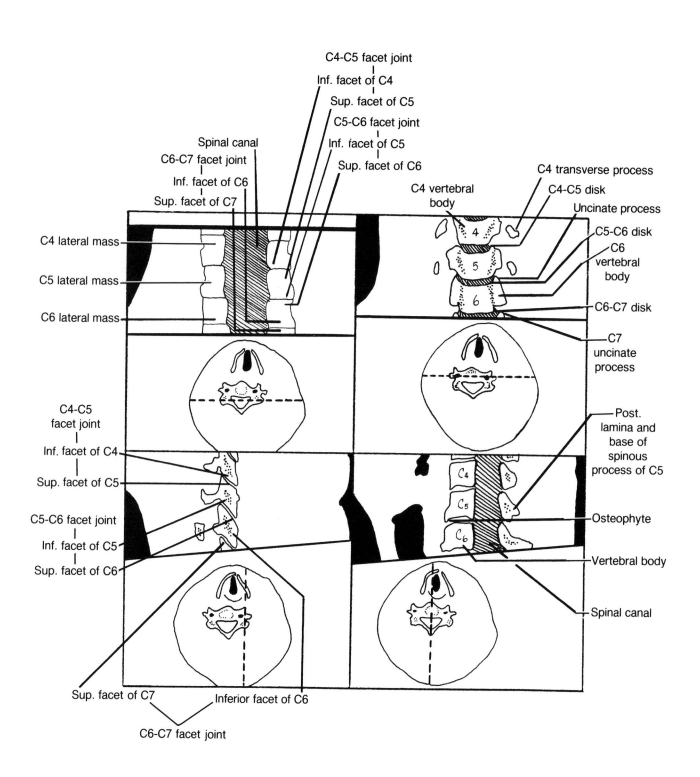

C4-C5 facet joint
Inf. facet of C4
Sup. facet of C5
C5-C6 facet joint
Inf. facet of C5
Sup. facet of C6

Spinal canal
C6-C7 facet joint
Inf. facet of C6
Sup. facet of C7

C4 vertebral body

C4 transverse process
C4-C5 disk
Uncinate process
C5-C6 disk
C6 vertebral body
C6-C7 disk
C7 uncinate process

C4 lateral mass
C5 lateral mass
C6 lateral mass

C4-C5 facet joint
Inf. facet of C4
Sup. facet of C5
C5-C6 facet joint
Inf. facet of C5
Sup. facet of C6

Post. lamina and base of spinous process of C5
Osteophyte
Vertebral body
Spinal canal

Sup. facet of C7
Inferior facet of C6
C6-C7 facet joint

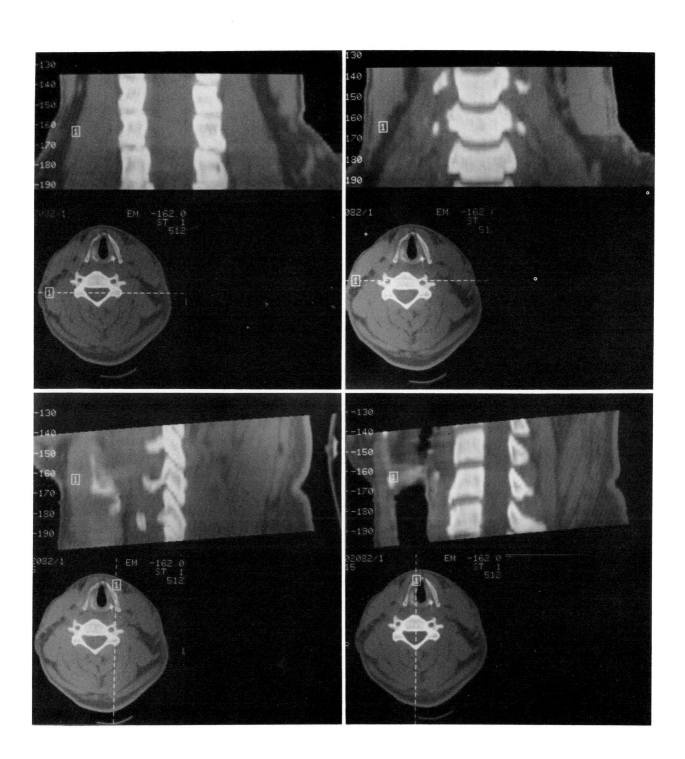

Thoracic Spine with Intrathecal Contrast

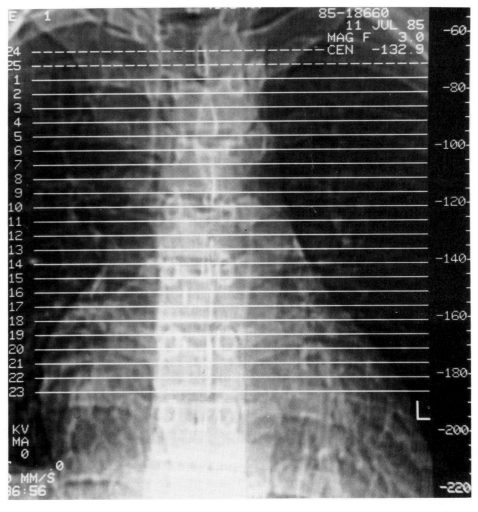

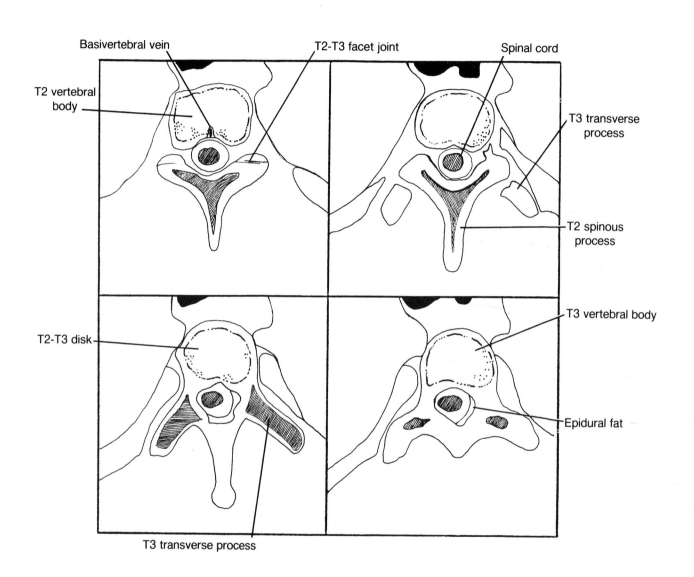

Basivertebral vein

T2-T3 facet joint

Spinal cord

T2 vertebral body

T3 transverse process

T2 spinous process

T2-T3 disk

T3 vertebral body

Epidural fat

T3 transverse process

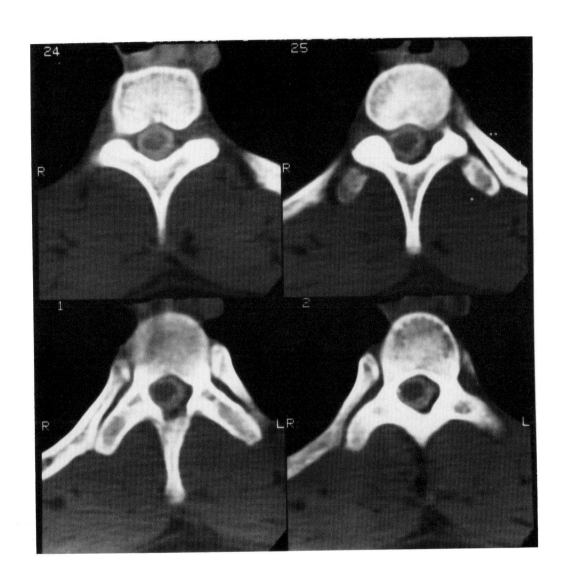

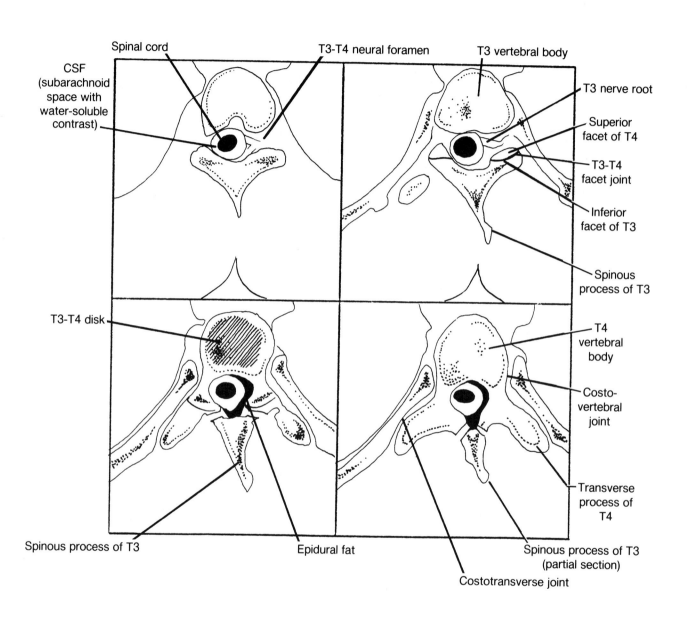

Spinal cord

T3-T4 neural foramen

T3 vertebral body

CSF (subarachnoid space with water-soluble contrast)

T3 nerve root

Superior facet of T4

T3-T4 facet joint

Inferior facet of T3

Spinous process of T3

T3-T4 disk

T4 vertebral body

Costo-vertebral joint

Transverse process of T4

Spinous process of T3

Epidural fat

Spinous process of T3 (partial section)

Costotransverse joint

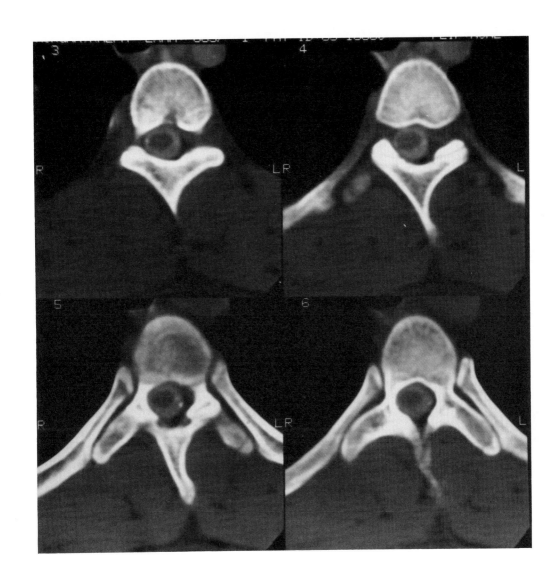

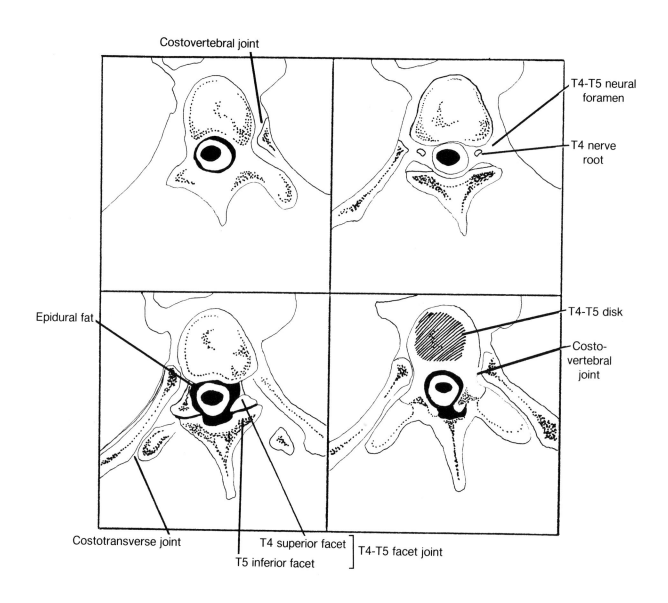

Costovertebral joint

T4-T5 neural foramen

T4 nerve root

Epidural fat

T4-T5 disk

Costovertebral joint

Costotransverse joint

T4 superior facet

T5 inferior facet

T4-T5 facet joint

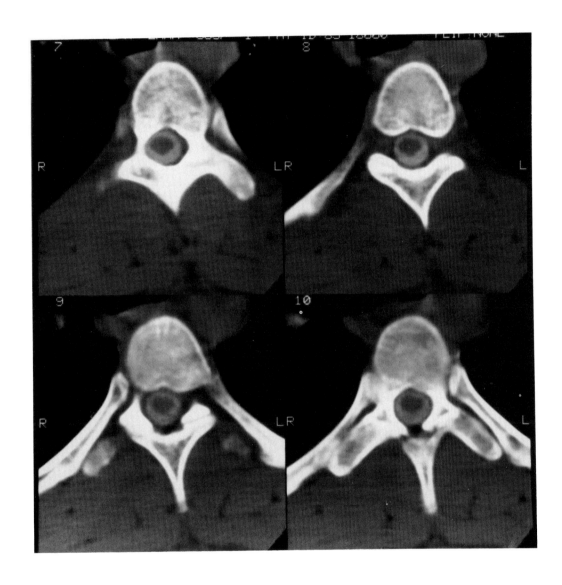

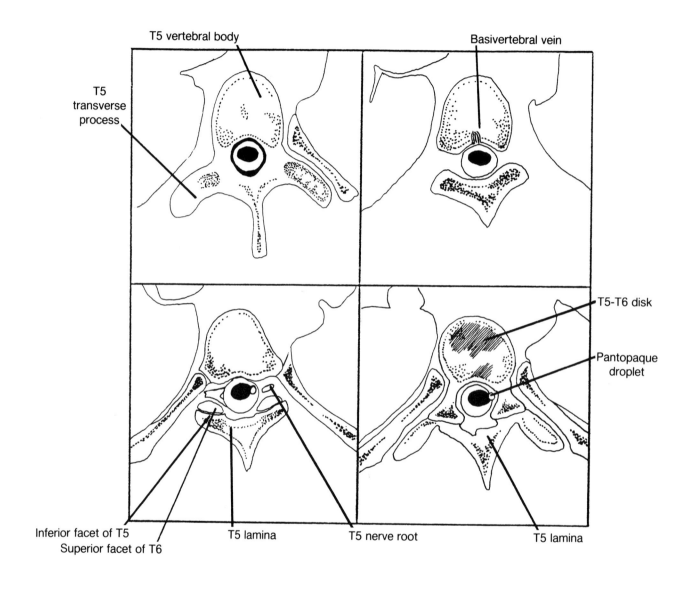

T5 vertebral body

Basivertebral vein

T5 transverse process

T5-T6 disk

Pantopaque droplet

Inferior facet of T5
Superior facet of T6

T5 lamina

T5 nerve root

T5 lamina

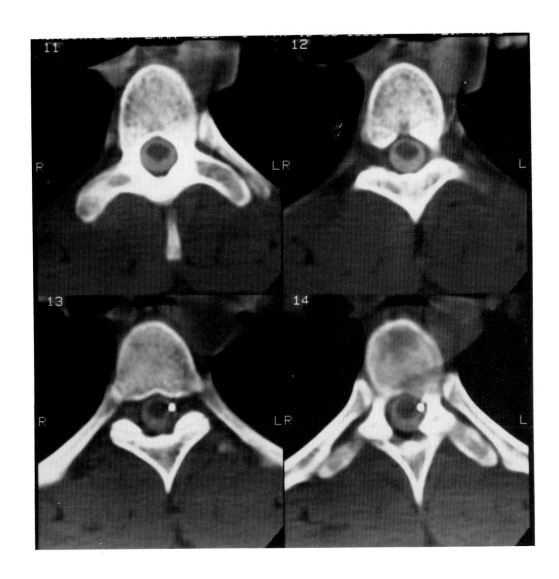

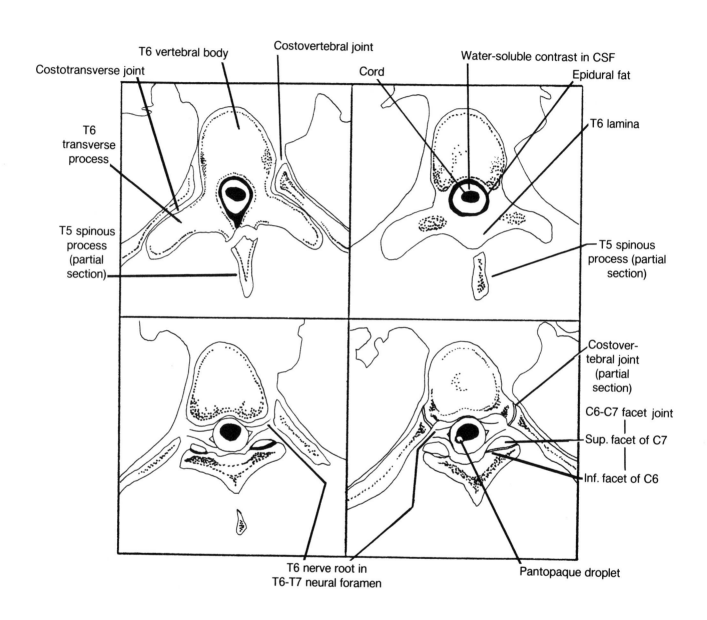

Costotransverse joint

T6 vertebral body

Costovertebral joint

Cord

Water-soluble contrast in CSF

Epidural fat

T6 transverse process

T6 lamina

T5 spinous process (partial section)

T5 spinous process (partial section)

Costover-tebral joint (partial section)

C6-C7 facet joint

Sup. facet of C7

Inf. facet of C6

T6 nerve root in T6-T7 neural foramen

Pantopaque droplet

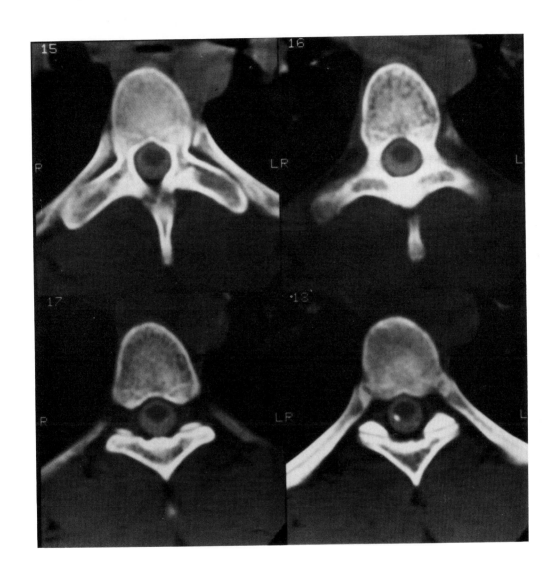

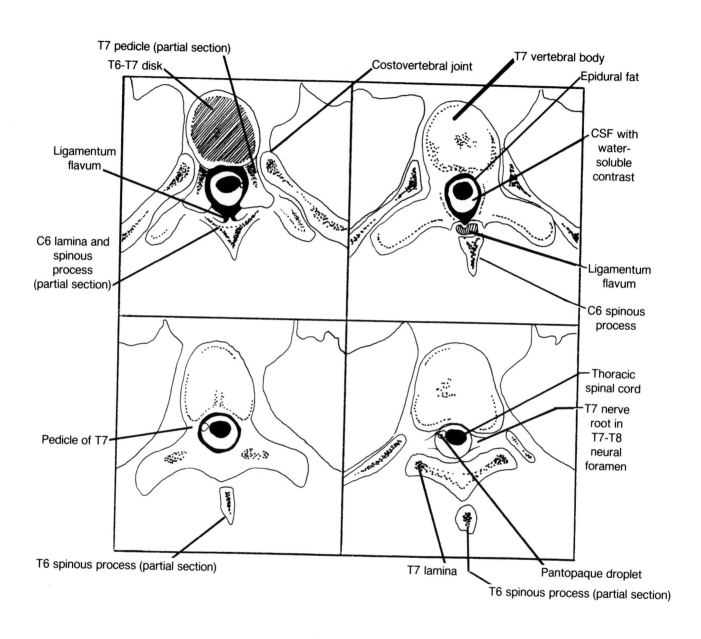

T7 pedicle (partial section)

T6-T7 disk

Costovertebral joint

T7 vertebral body

Epidural fat

Ligamentum flavum

CSF with water-soluble contrast

C6 lamina and spinous process (partial section)

Ligamentum flavum

C6 spinous process

Pedicle of T7

Thoracic spinal cord

T7 nerve root in T7-T8 neural foramen

T6 spinous process (partial section)

T7 lamina

Pantopaque droplet

T6 spinous process (partial section)

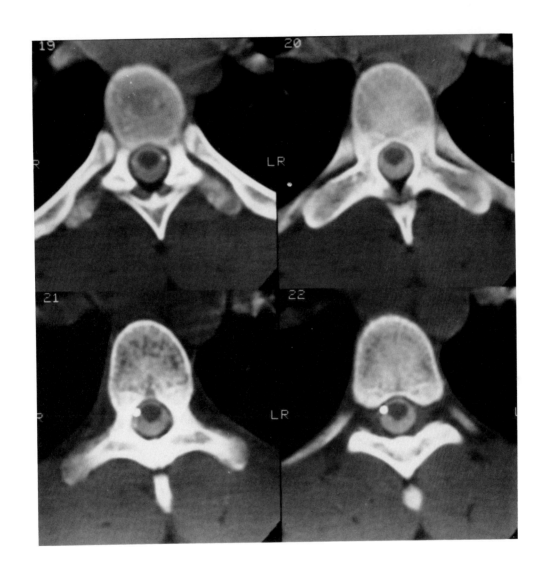

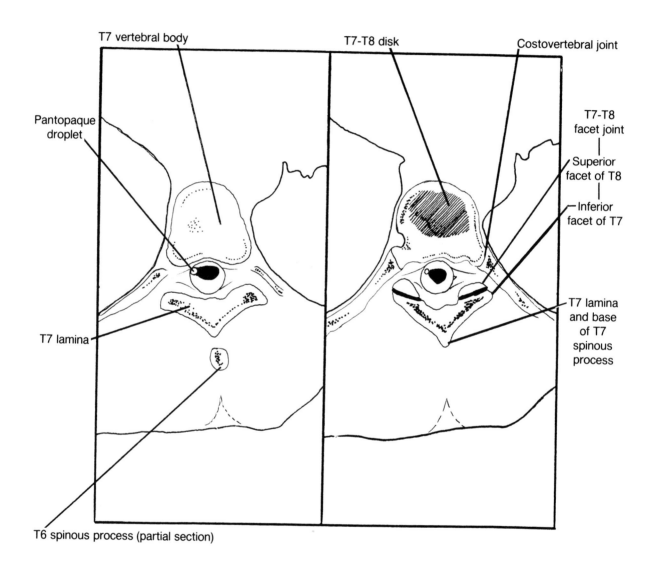

T7 vertebral body

T7-T8 disk

Costovertebral joint

Pantopaque
droplet

T7-T8
facet joint

Superior
facet of T8

Inferior
facet of T7

T7 lamina

T7 lamina
and base
of T7
spinous
process

T6 spinous process (partial section)

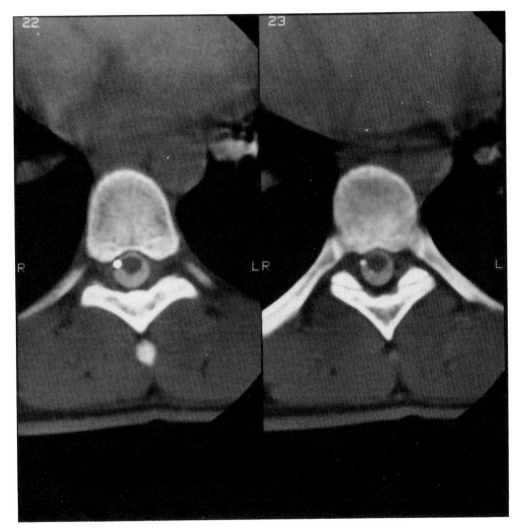

Image 22 is repeated from p 325.

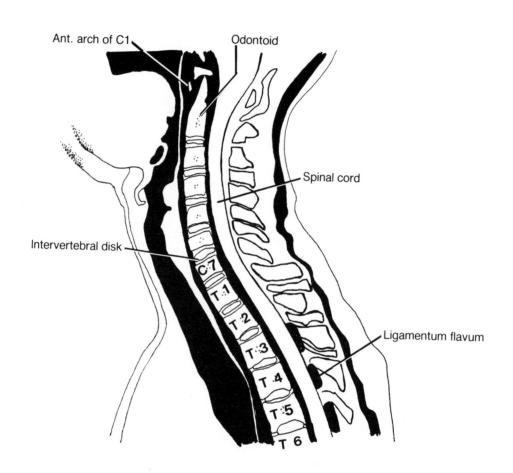

Ant. arch of C1

Odontoid

Spinal cord

Intervertebral disk

Ligamentum flavum

C 7
T 1
T 2
T 3
T 4
T 5
T 6

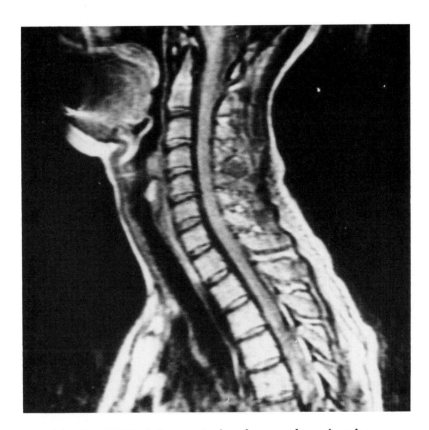

Midsagittal MRI of the cervical and upper thoracic spine.

Conus
Medullaris with
Intrathecal
Contrast

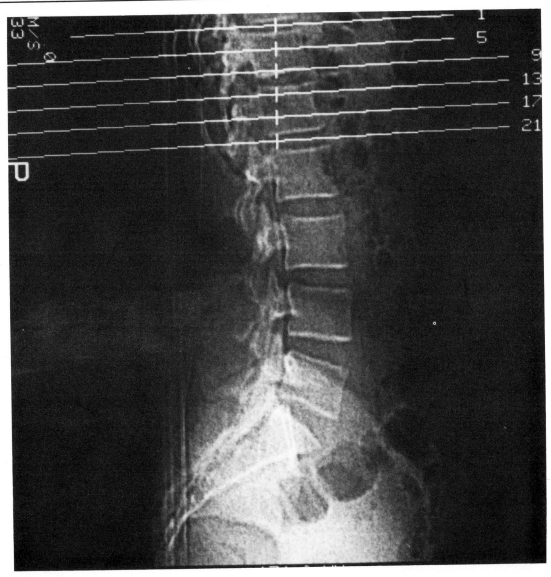

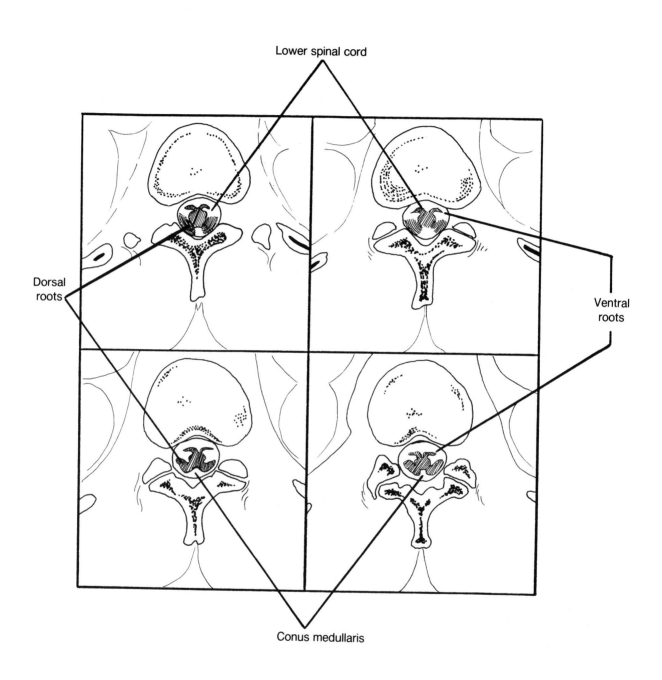

Lower spinal cord

Dorsal roots

Ventral roots

Conus medullaris

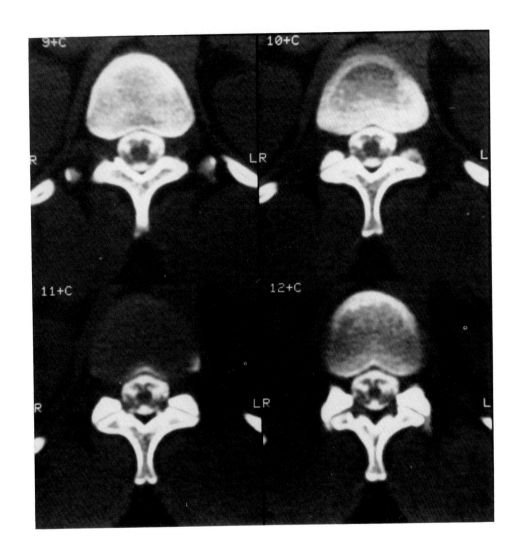

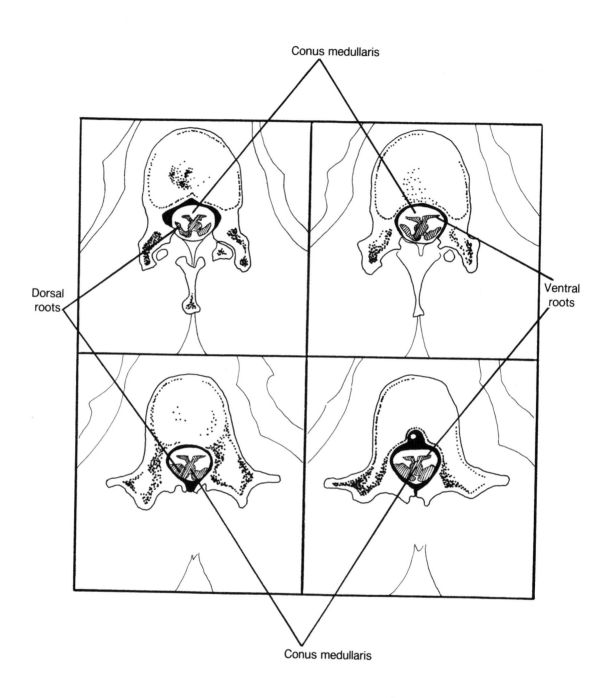

Conus medullaris

Dorsal roots

Ventral roots

Conus medullaris

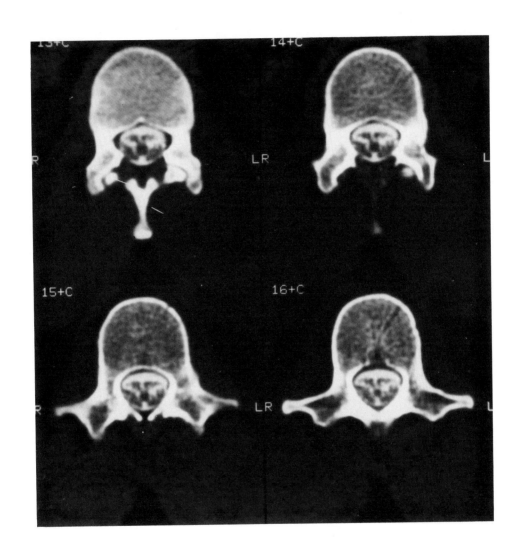

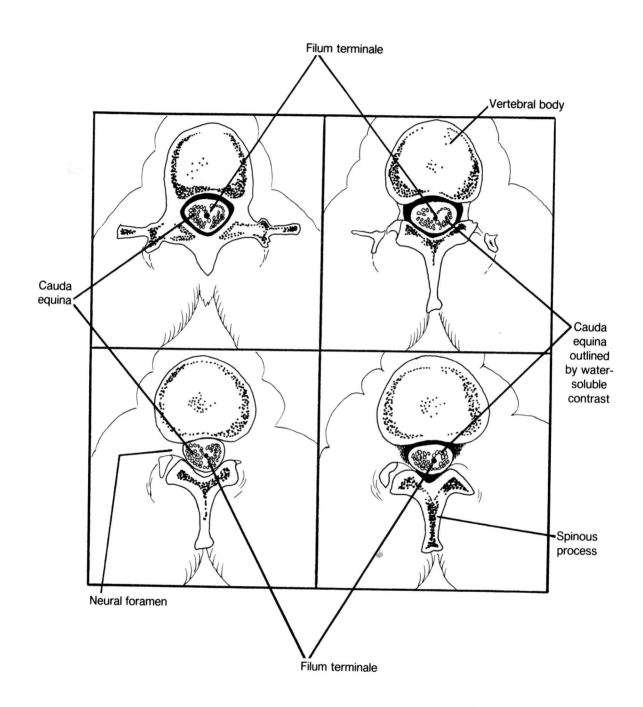

Filum terminale

Vertebral body

Cauda equina

Cauda equina outlined by water-soluble contrast

Neural foramen

Spinous process

Filum terminale

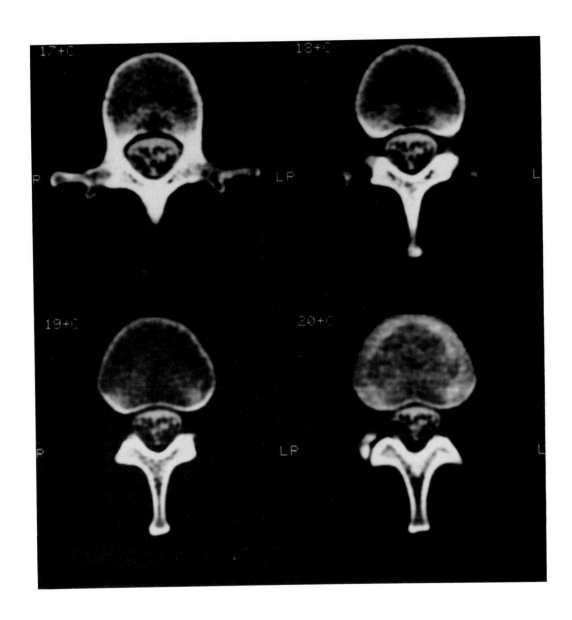

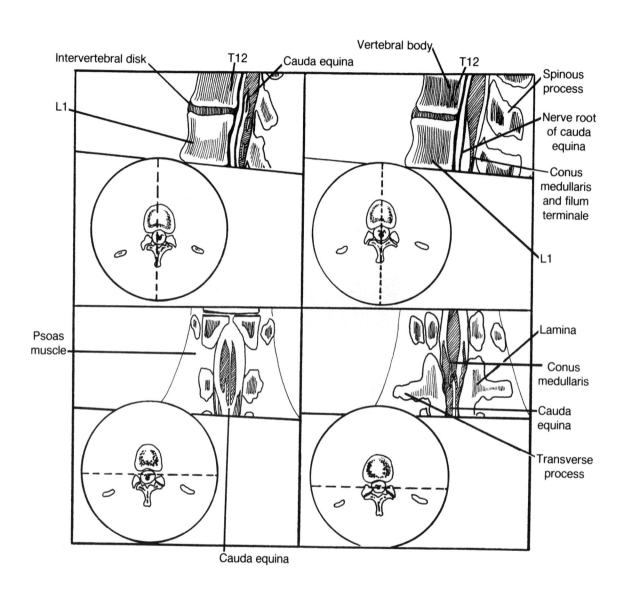

Intervertebral disk

T12

Cauda equina

Vertebral body

T12

Spinous process

Nerve root of cauda equina

Conus medullaris and filum terminale

L1

L1

Psoas muscle

Lamina

Conus medullaris

Cauda equina

Transverse process

Cauda equina

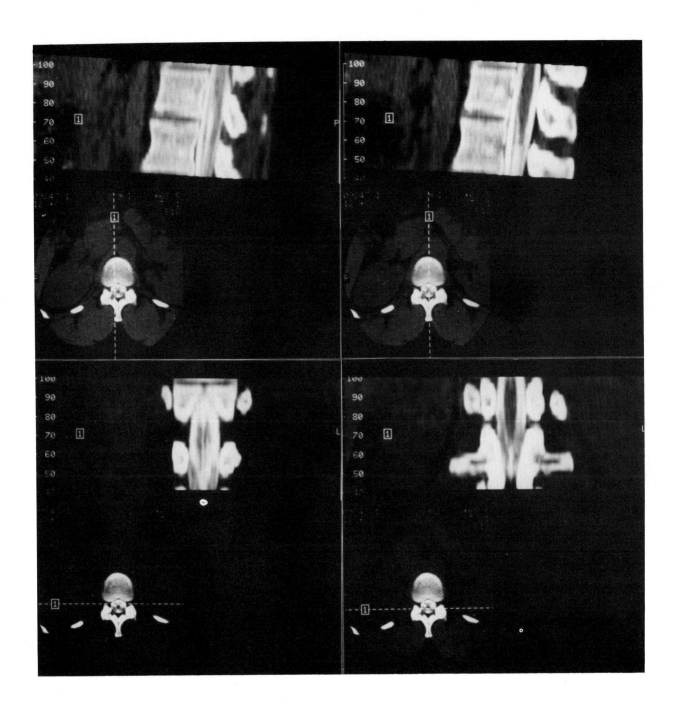

Lumbosacral Spine: L3-L4 without Intrathecal Contrast

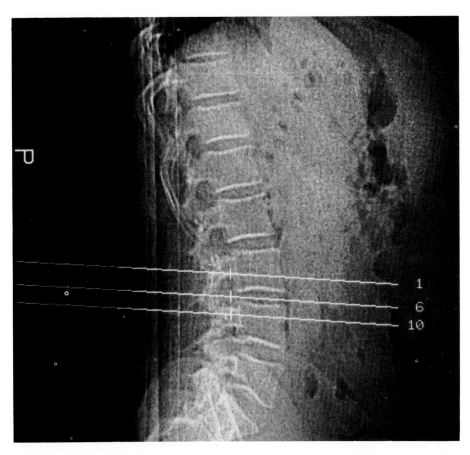

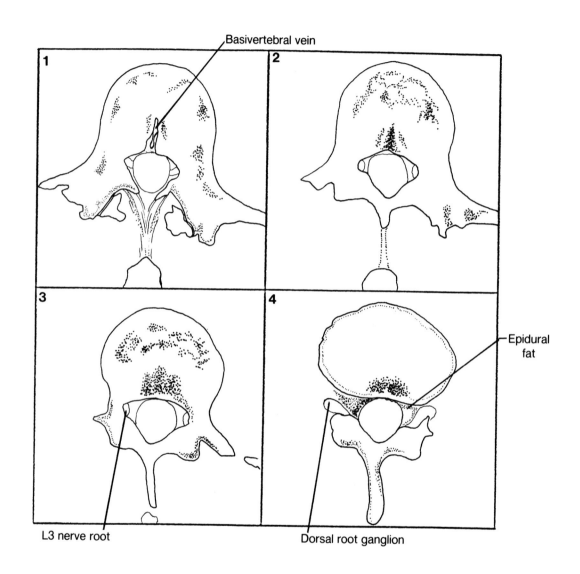

Basivertebral vein

Epidural fat

L3 nerve root

Dorsal root ganglion

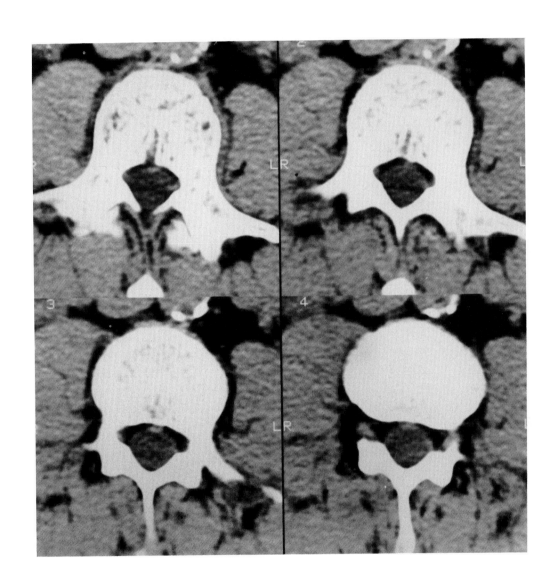

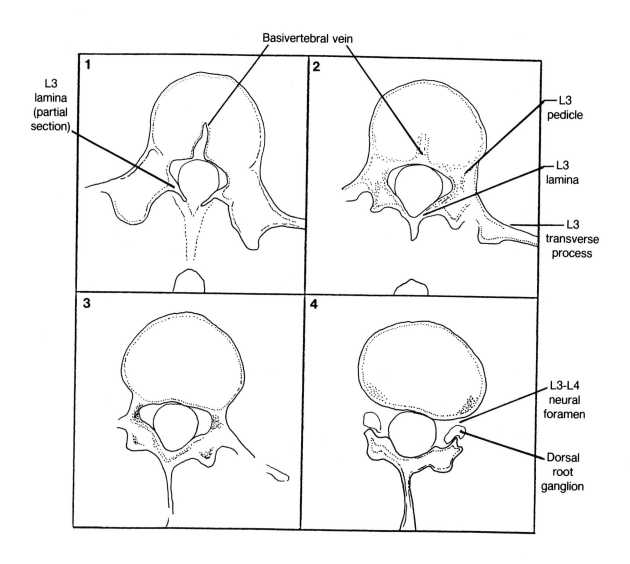

Basivertebral vein

1

L3
lamina
(partial
section)

2

L3
pedicle

L3
lamina

L3
transverse
process

3

4

L3-L4
neural
foramen

Dorsal
root
ganglion

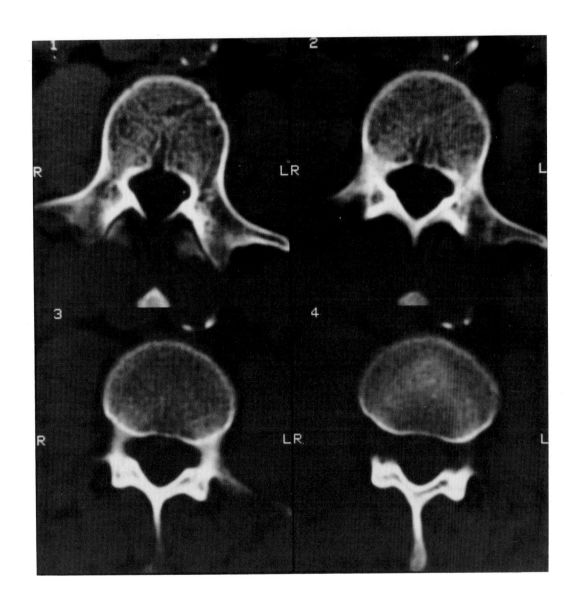

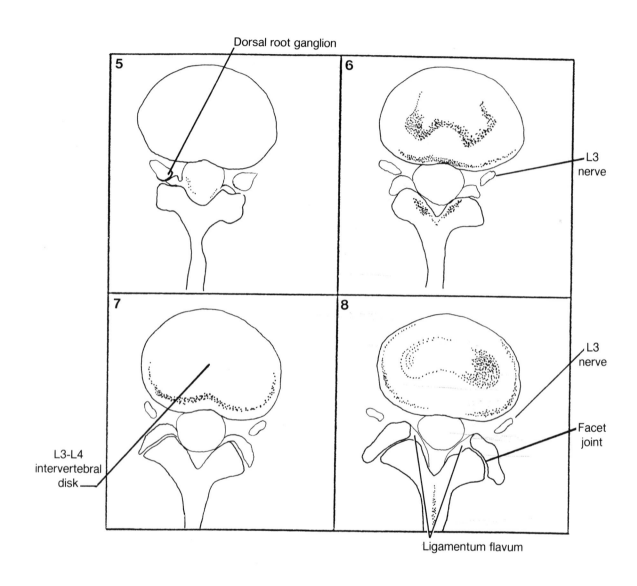

Dorsal root ganglion

5

6

L3
nerve

7

8

L3
nerve

Facet
joint

L3-L4
intervertebral
disk

Ligamentum flavum

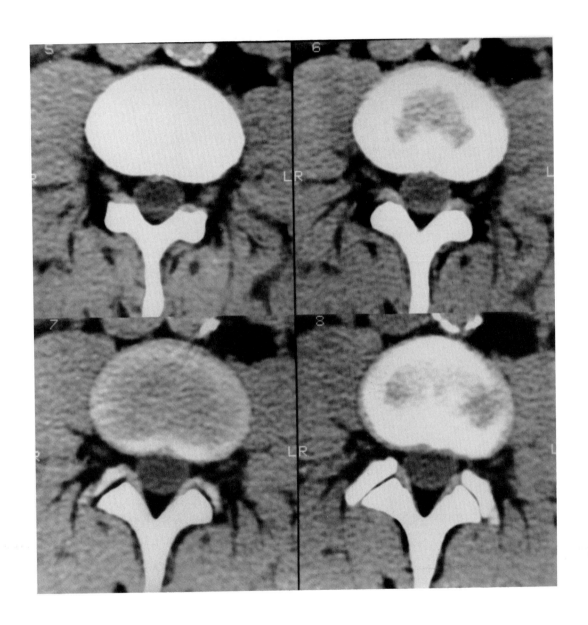

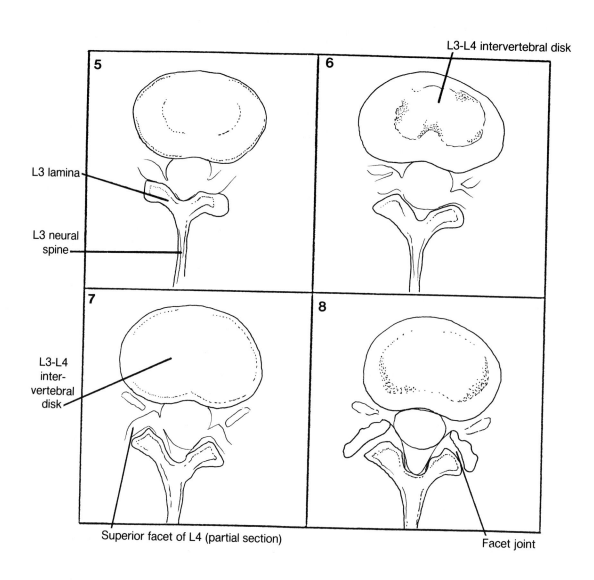

5

6

L3-L4 intervertebral disk

L3 lamina

L3 neural spine

7

L3-L4 inter-vertebral disk

8

Superior facet of L4 (partial section)

Facet joint

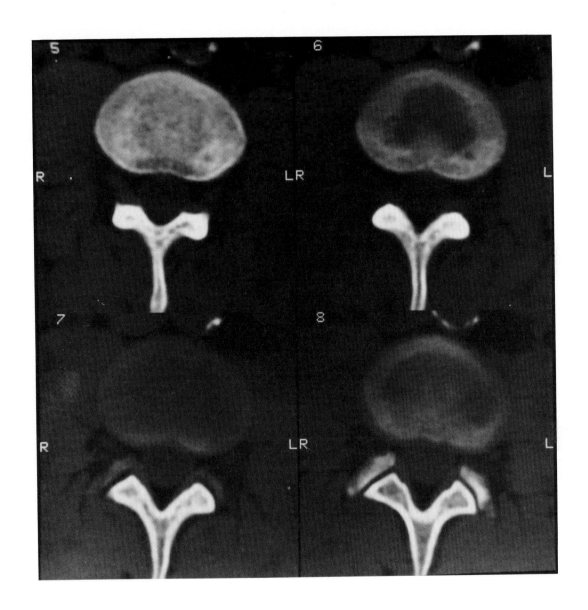

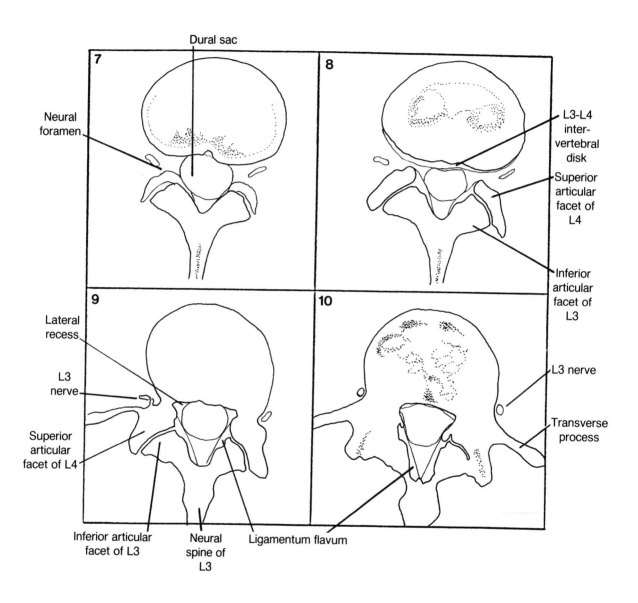

Dural sac

7

Neural
foramen

8

L3-L4
inter-
vertebral
disk

Superior
articular
facet of
L4

Inferior
articular
facet of
L3

9

Lateral
recess

L3
nerve

Superior
articular
facet of L4

10

L3 nerve

Transverse
process

Inferior articular
facet of L3

Neural
spine of
L3

Ligamentum flavum

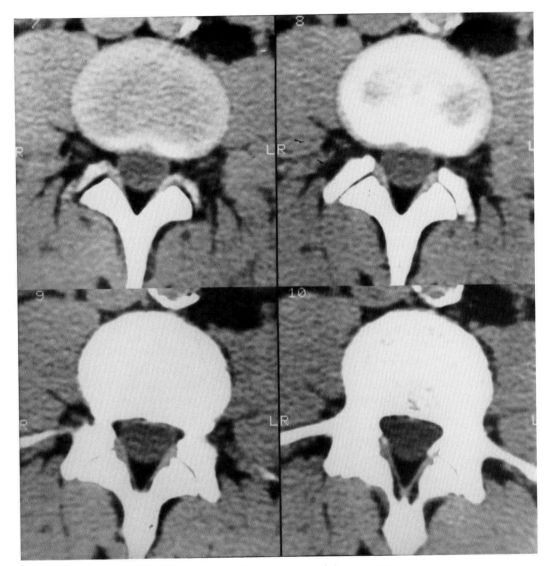

Images 7 and 8 are repeated from p 347.

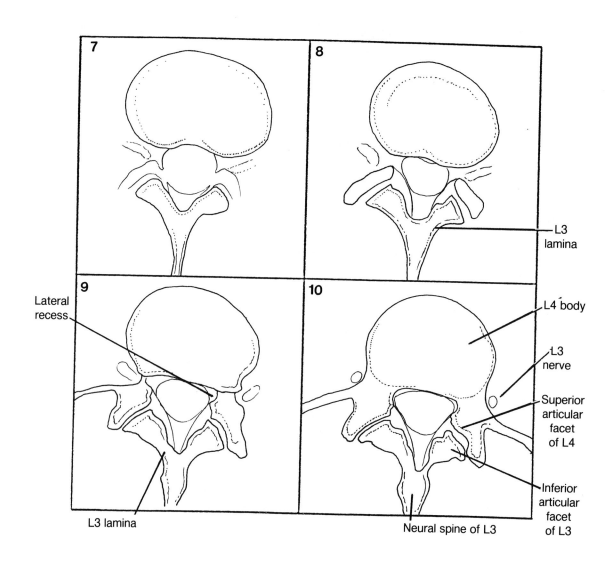

7

8
L3
lamina

9
Lateral
recess

L3 lamina

10
L4 body

L3
nerve

Superior
articular
facet
of L4

Inferior
articular
facet
of L3

Neural spine of L3

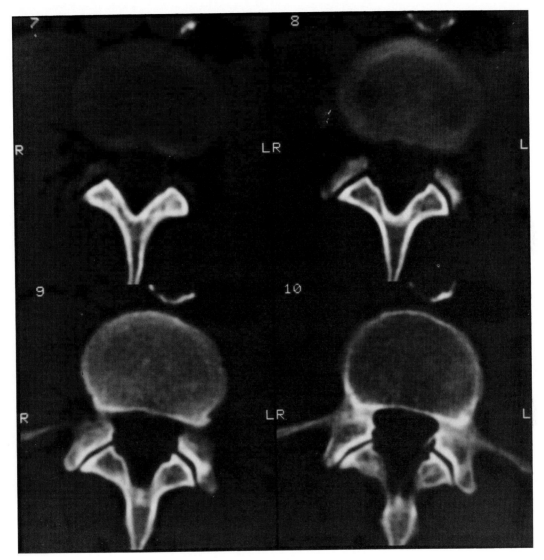

Images 7 and 8 are repeated from p 349.

Lumbosacral Spine: L4-L5 without Intrathecal Contrast

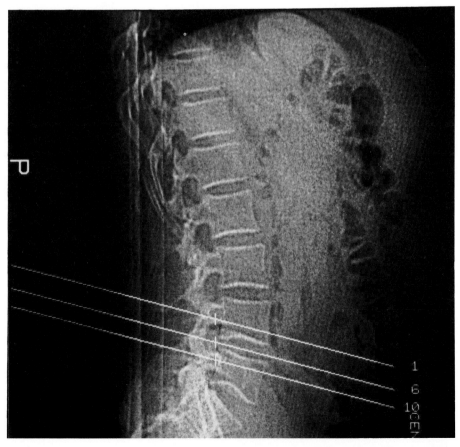

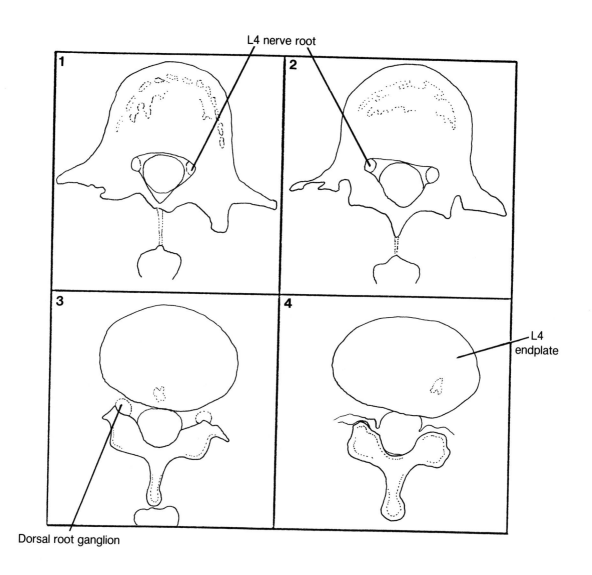

L4 nerve root

L4 endplate

Dorsal root ganglion

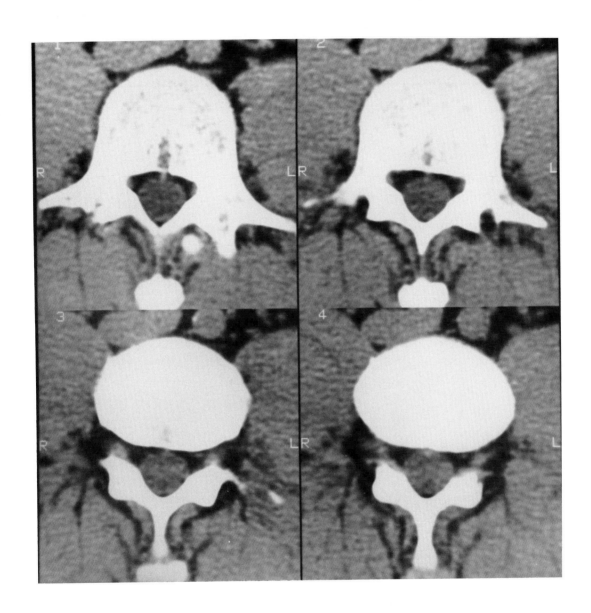

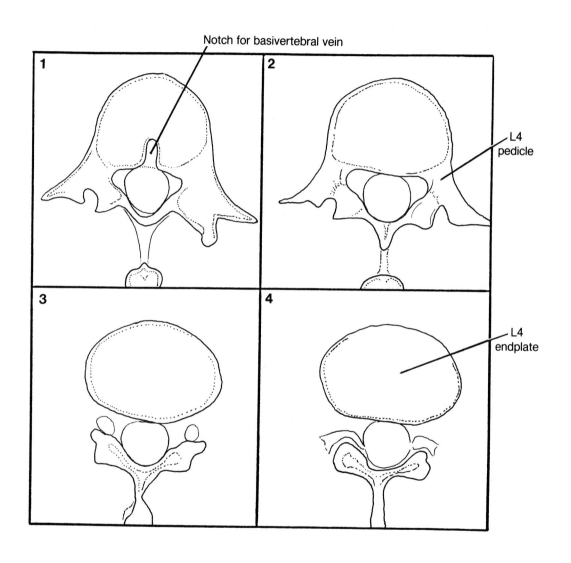

Notch for basivertebral vein

L4 pedicle

L4 endplate

Lumbosacral Spine: L5-S1 without Intrathecal Contrast

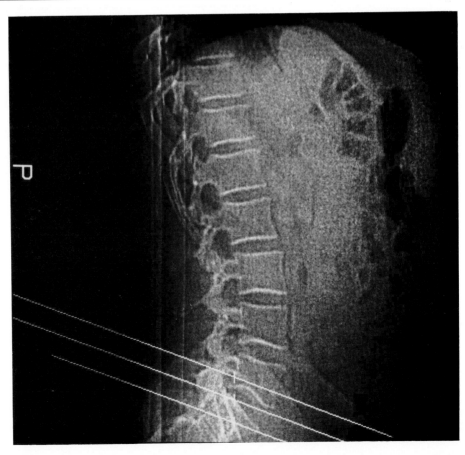

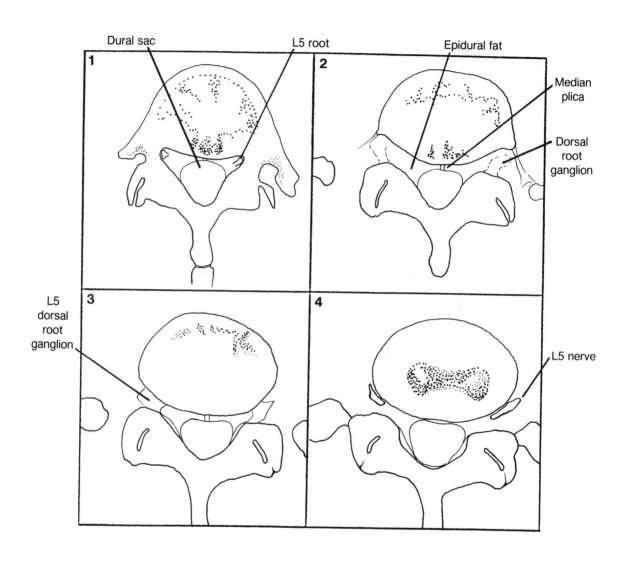

Dural sac

L5 root

Epidural fat

Median plica

Dorsal root ganglion

L5 dorsal root ganglion

L5 nerve

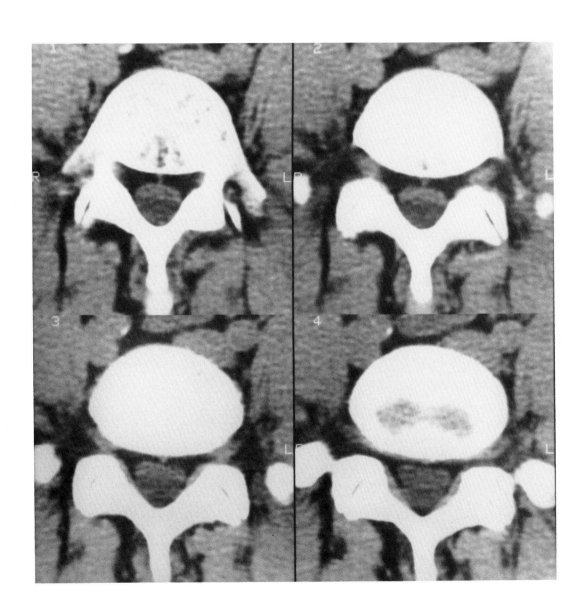

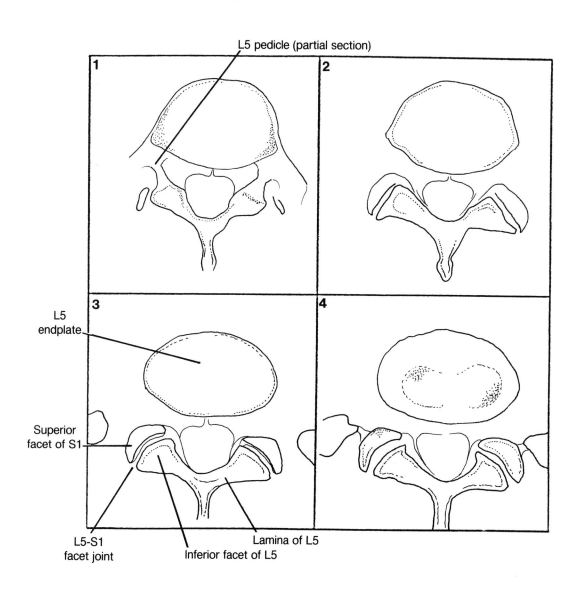

L5 pedicle (partial section)

L5 endplate

Superior facet of S1

L5-S1 facet joint

Inferior facet of L5

Lamina of L5

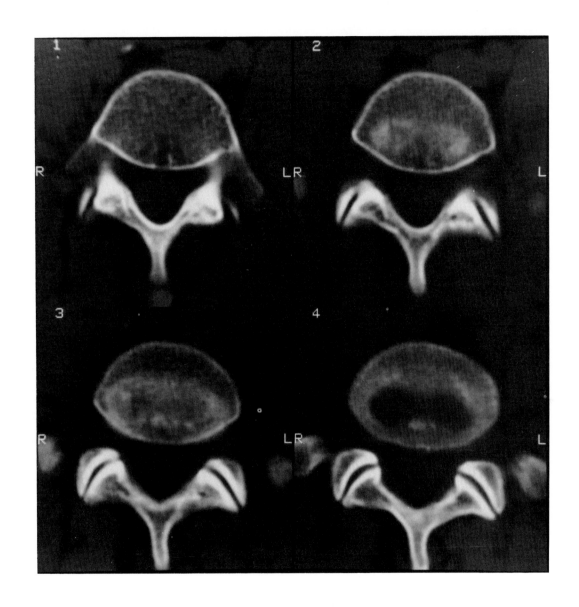

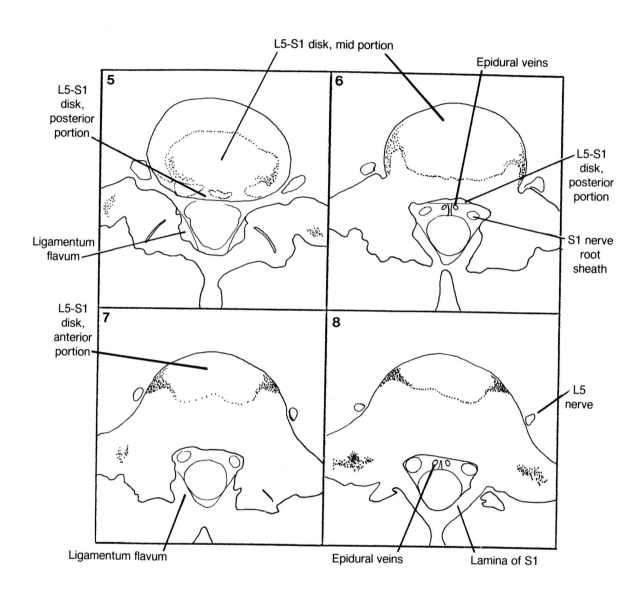

L5-S1 disk, mid portion

Epidural veins

L5-S1 disk, posterior portion

L5-S1 disk, posterior portion

Ligamentum flavum

S1 nerve root sheath

L5-S1 disk, anterior portion

L5 nerve

Ligamentum flavum

Epidural veins

Lamina of S1

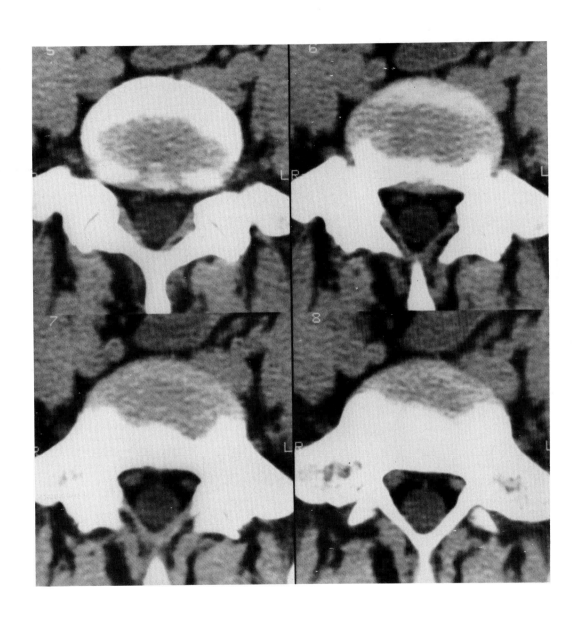

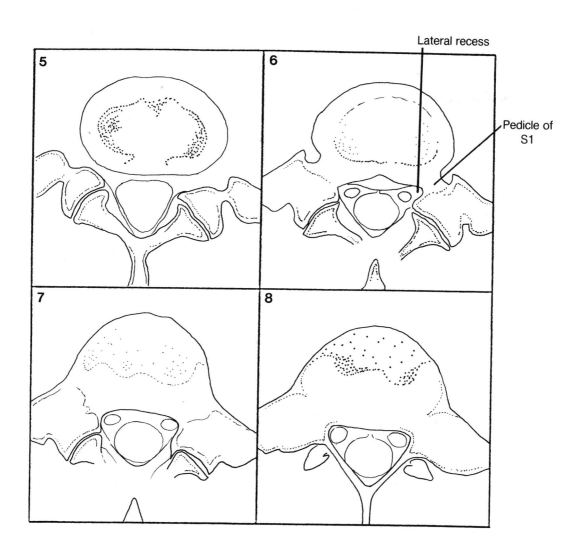

Lateral recess

Pedicle of
S1

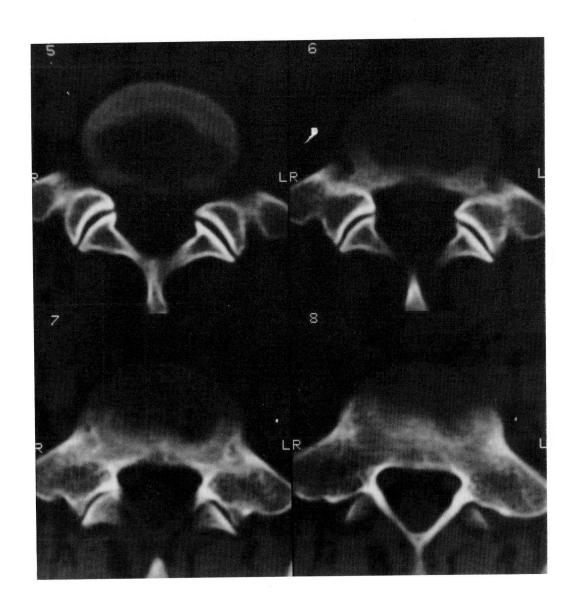

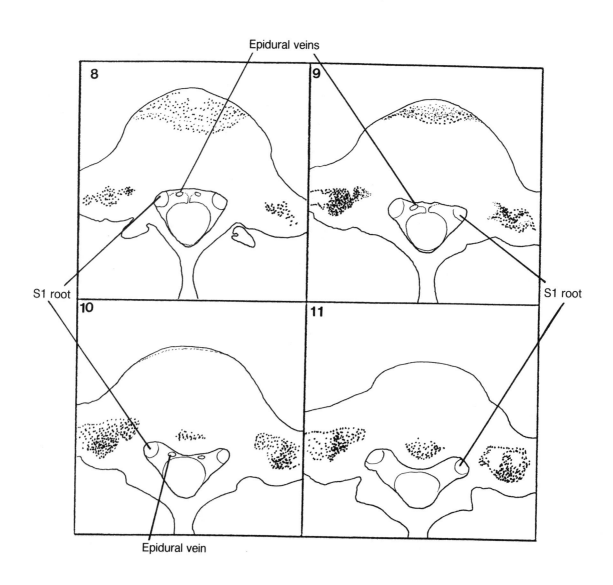

Epidural veins

8

9

S1 root

S1 root

10

11

Epidural vein

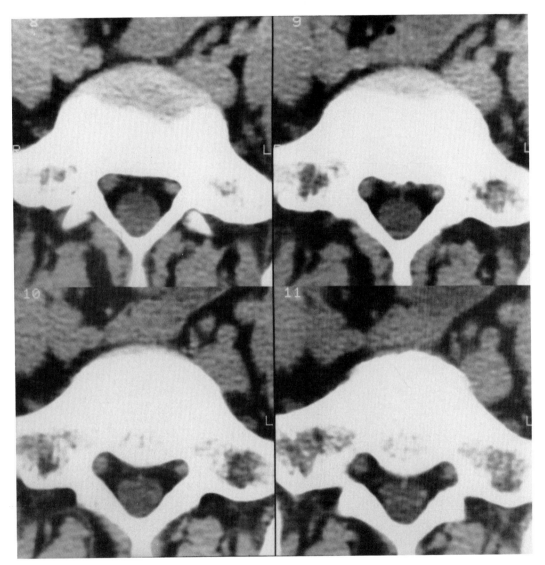

Image 8 is repeated from p 375.

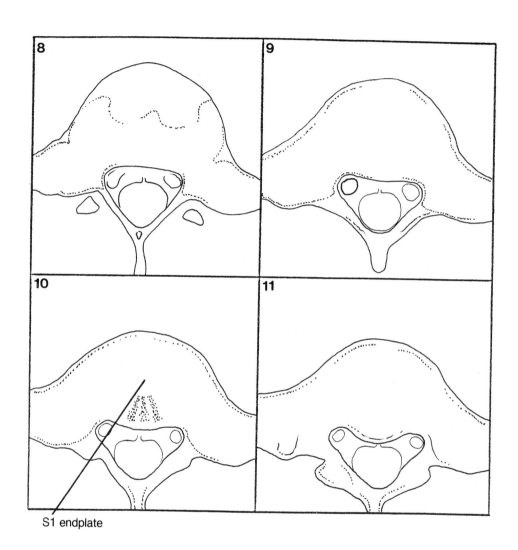

S1 endplate

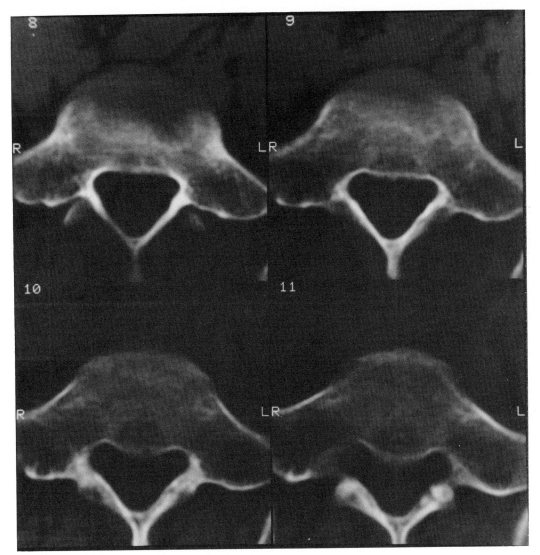

Image 8 is repeated from p 377.

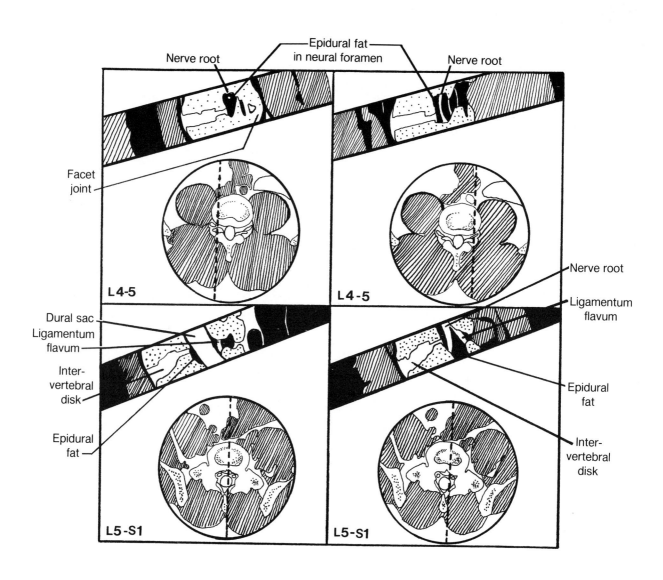

Nerve root

Epidural fat
in neural foramen

Nerve root

Facet
joint

L4-5

L4-5

Nerve root

Ligamentum
flavum

Dural sac

Ligamentum
flavum

Inter-
vertebral
disk

Epidural
fat

Inter-
vertebral
disk

Epidural
fat

L5-S1

L5-S1

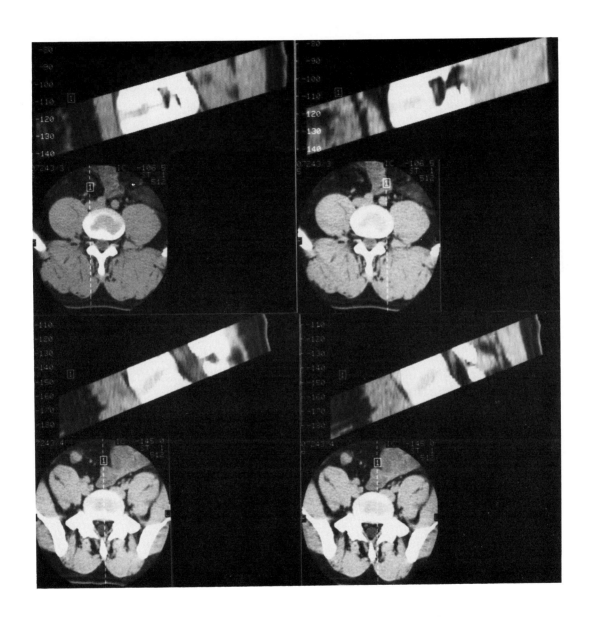

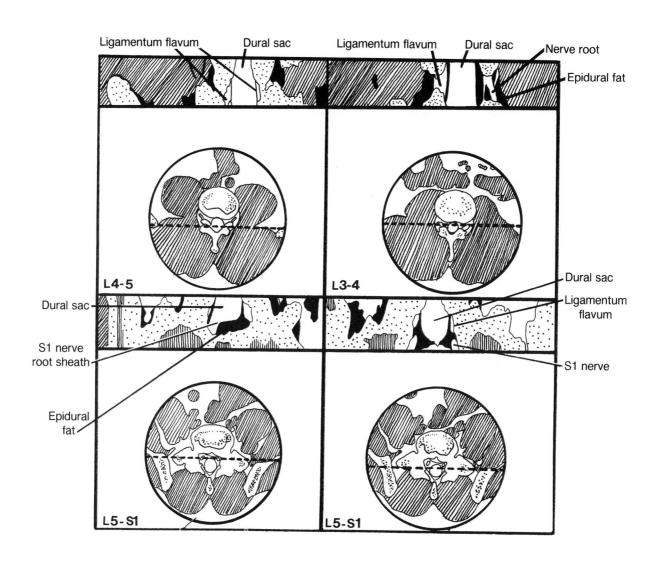

Ligamentum flavum   Dural sac   Ligamentum flavum   Dural sac   Nerve root

Epidural fat

L4-5   L3-4

Dural sac   Dural sac

Ligamentum flavum

S1 nerve root sheath   S1 nerve

Epidural fat

L5-S1   L5-S1

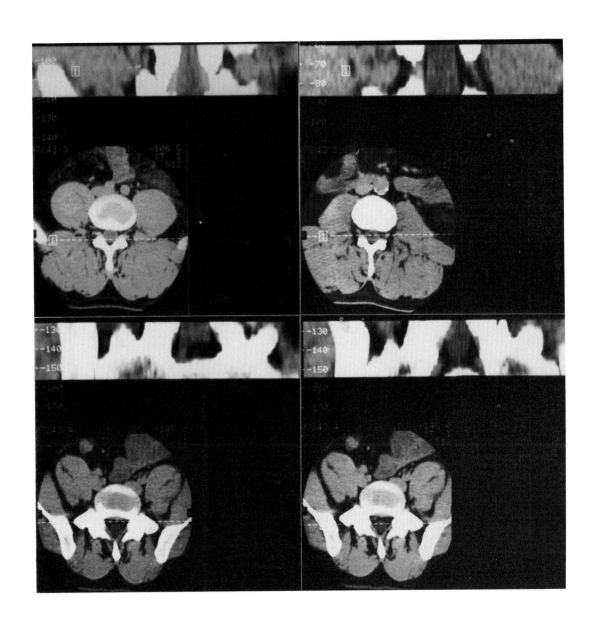

Lumbosacral Spine: L5-S1 with Intrathecal Contrast

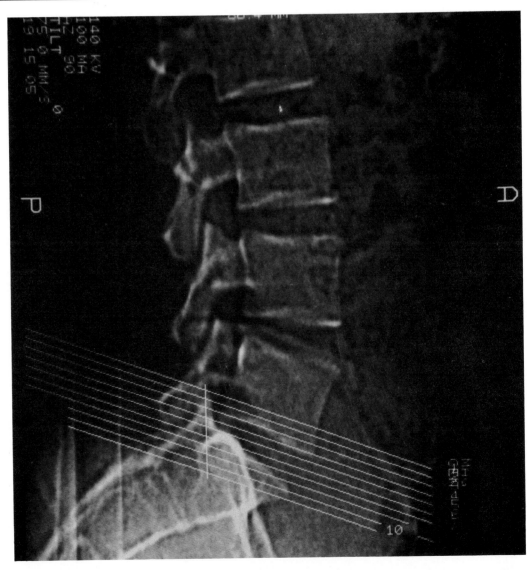

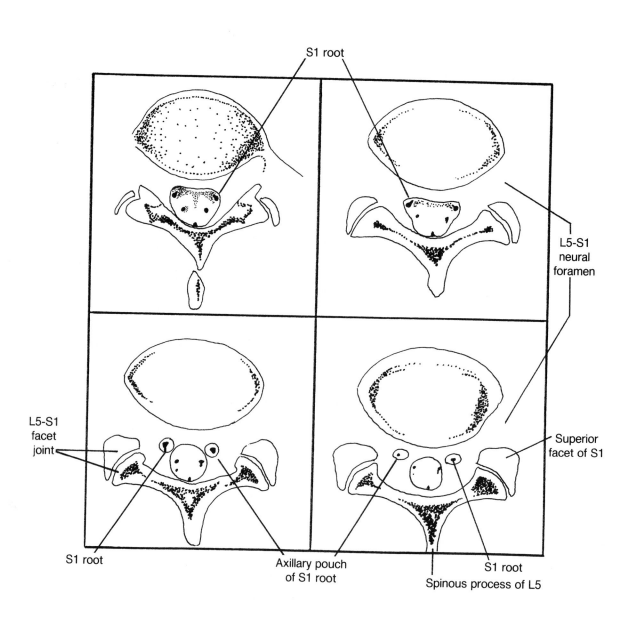

S1 root

L5-S1
neural
foramen

L5-S1
facet
joint

Superior
facet of S1

S1 root

Axillary pouch
of S1 root

S1 root

Spinous process of L5

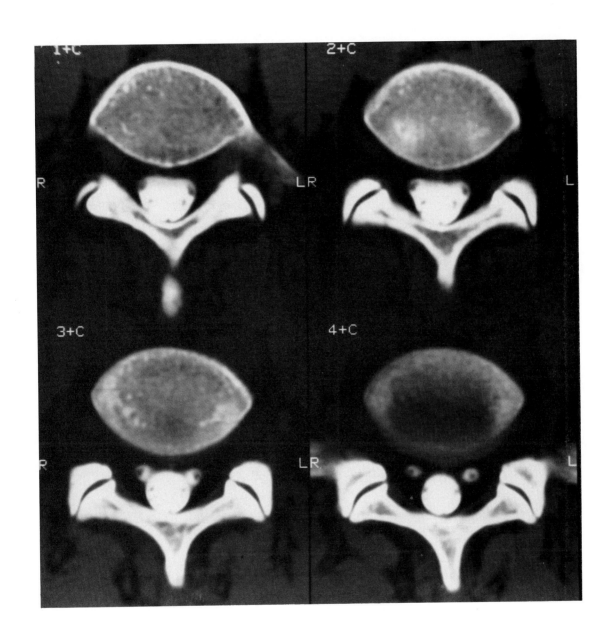

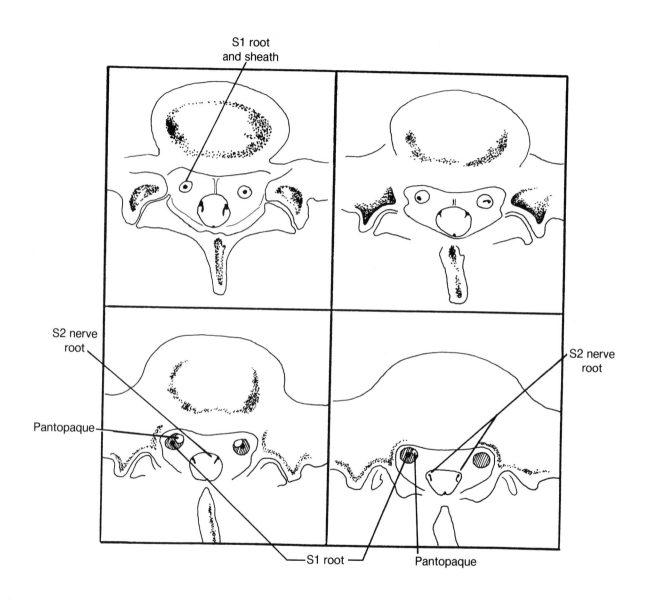

S1 root
and sheath

S2 nerve
root

Pantopaque

S2 nerve
root

S1 root

Pantopaque

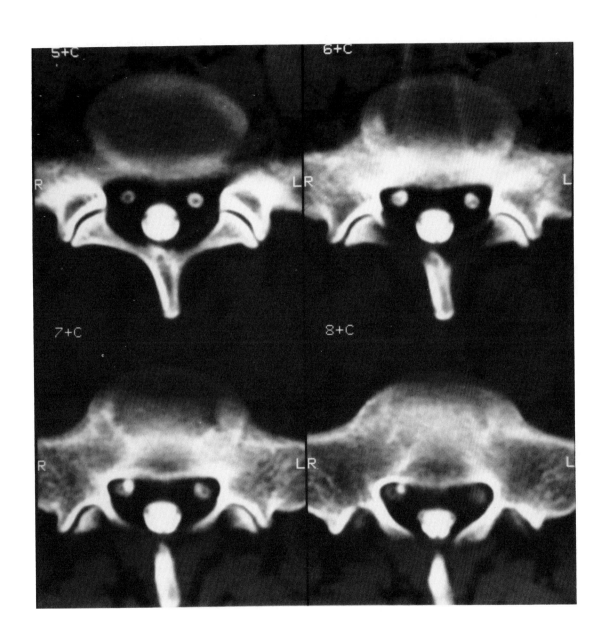

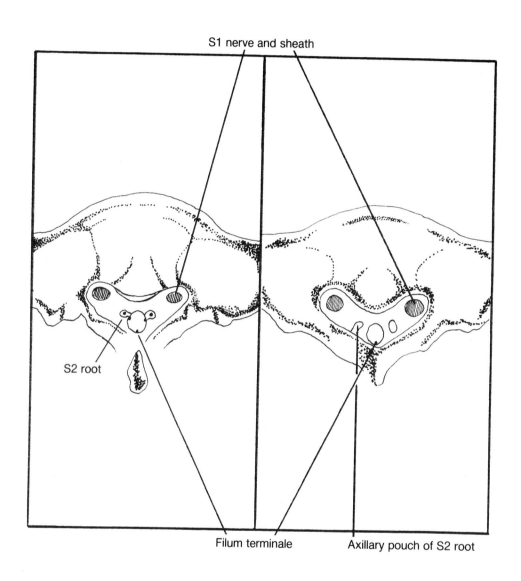

S1 nerve and sheath

S2 root

Filum terminale

Axillary pouch of S2 root

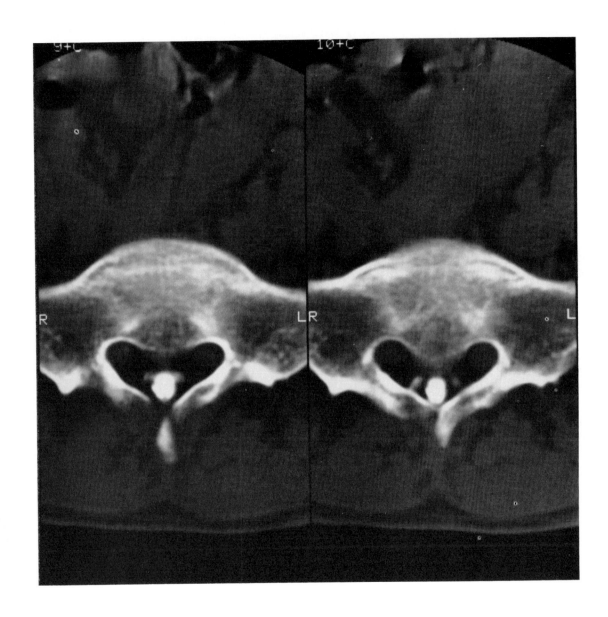

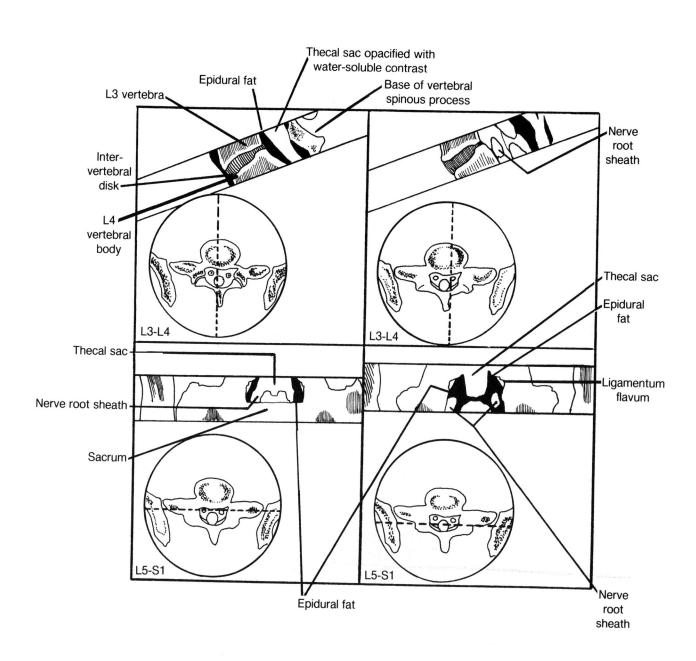

Thecal sac opacified with
water-soluble contrast

Epidural fat

L3 vertebra

Base of vertebral
spinous process

Inter-
vertebral
disk

Nerve
root
sheath

L4
vertebral
body

Thecal sac

Epidural
fat

L3-L4

L3-L4

Thecal sac

Ligamentum
flavum

Nerve root sheath

Sacrum

L5-S1

L5-S1

Epidural fat

Nerve
root
sheath

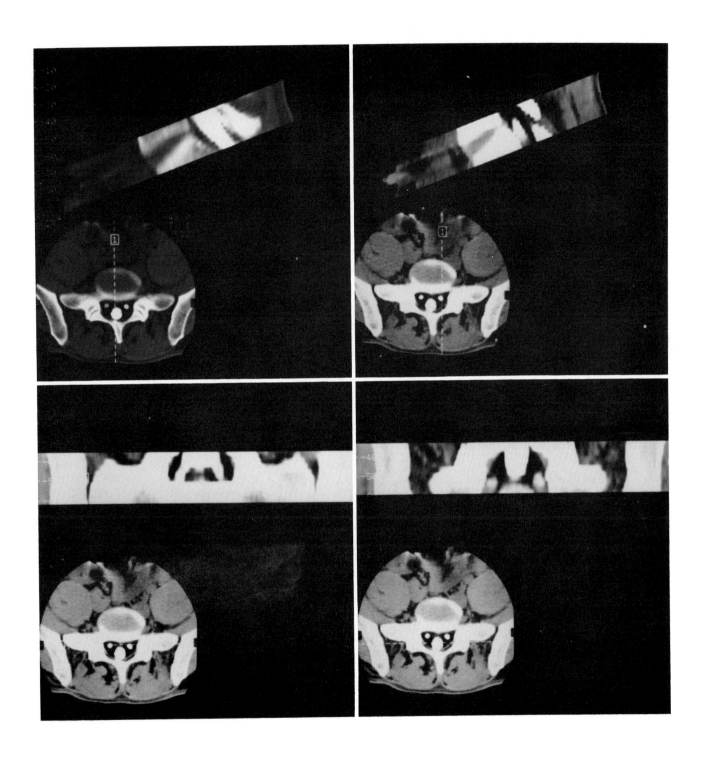

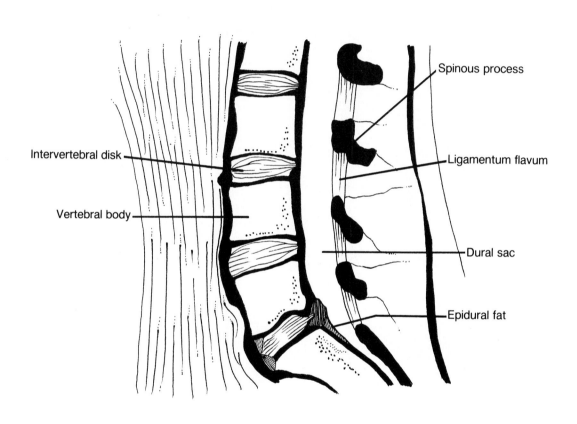

Intervertebral disk

Vertebral body

Spinous process

Ligamentum flavum

Dural sac

Epidural fat

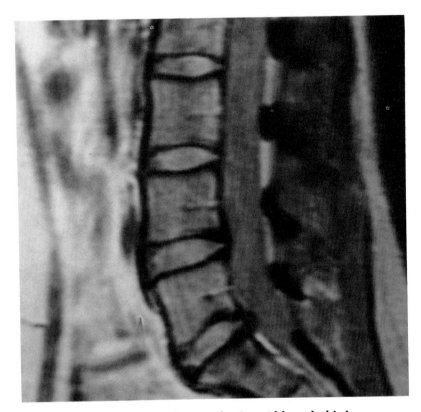

Midsagittal MRI of the lumbosacral spine. Although this image was obtained from an asymptomatic volunteer, the findings at L5-S1 suggest disk protrusion.

7 Neck

NASOPHARYNX
OROPHARYNX
HYPOPHARYNX AND LARYNX
LOWER NECK

This chapter illustrates the neck from the base of the skull to the thoracic inlet. CT slices are usually obtained at 5-mm intervals with 5-mm thickness. The patient is asked to breathe quietly so that the vocal cords are abducted and the glottis is open during the radiographic exposure. Selected levels are displayed here, using soft tissue and bone windows.

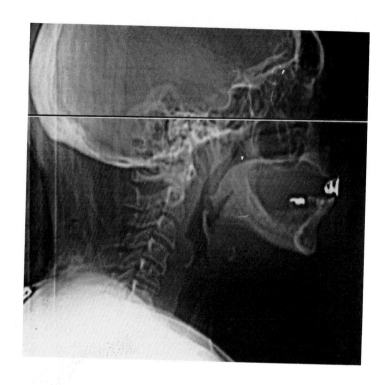

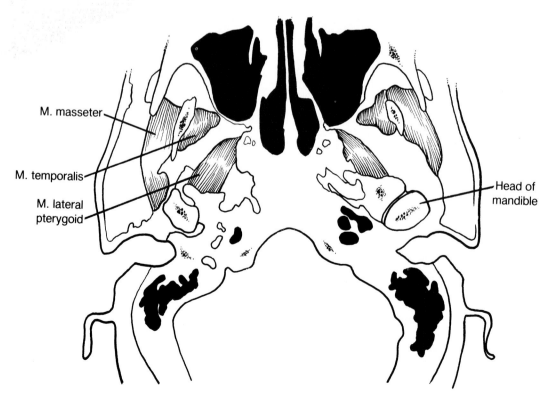

M. masseter

M. temporalis

M. lateral
pterygoid

Head of
mandible

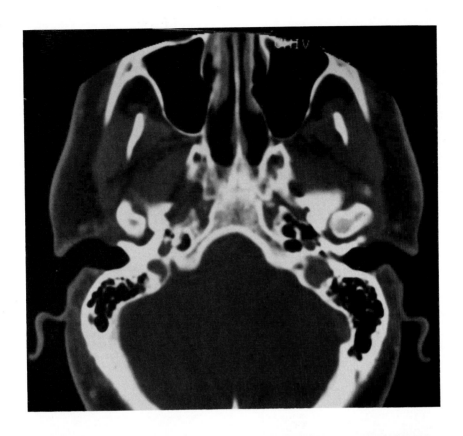

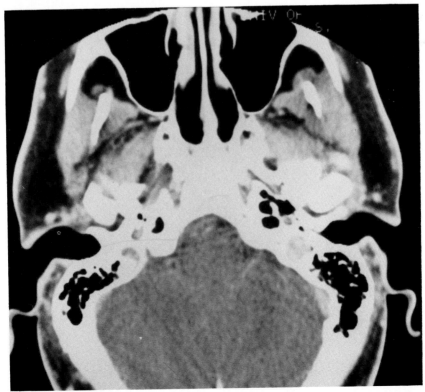

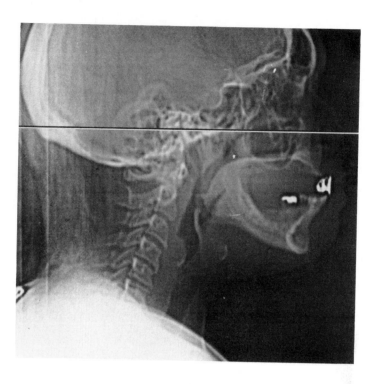

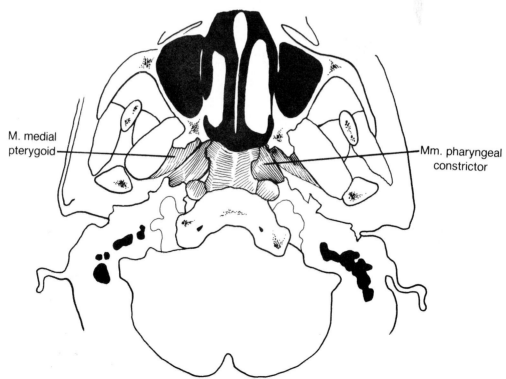

M. medial
pterygoid

Mm. pharyngeal
constrictor

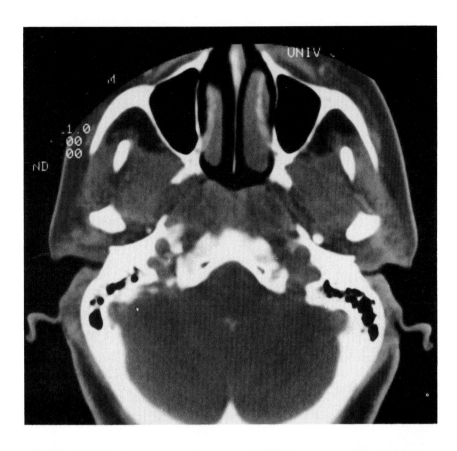

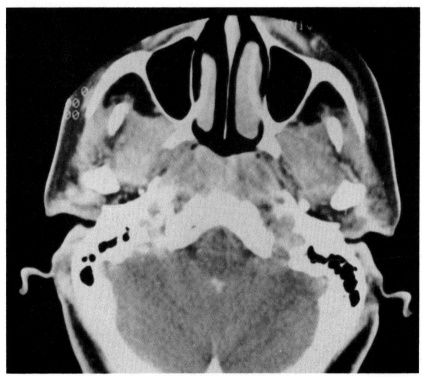

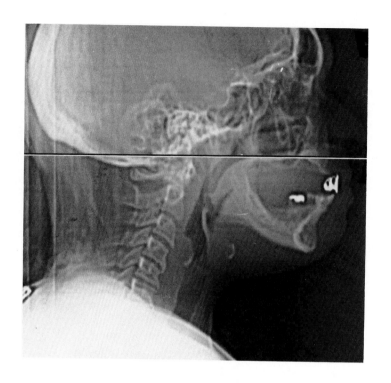

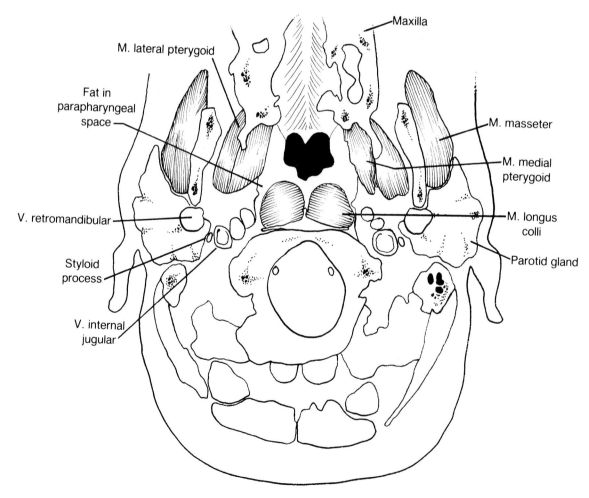

Maxilla

M. lateral pterygoid

Fat in
parapharyngeal
space

M. masseter

M. medial
pterygoid

V. retromandibular

M. longus
colli

Styloid
process

Parotid gland

V. internal
jugular

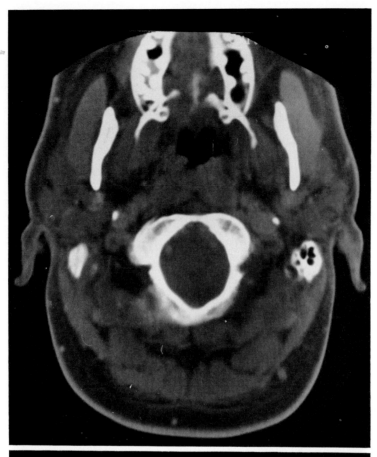

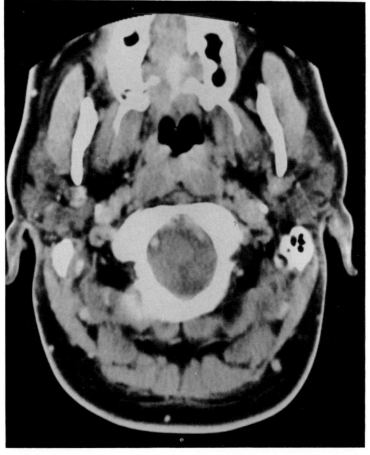

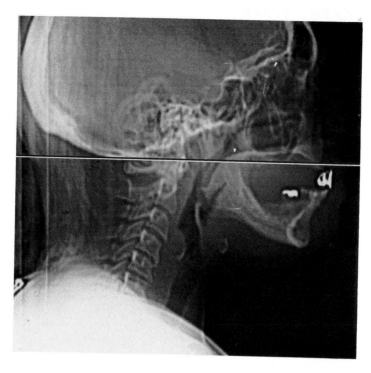

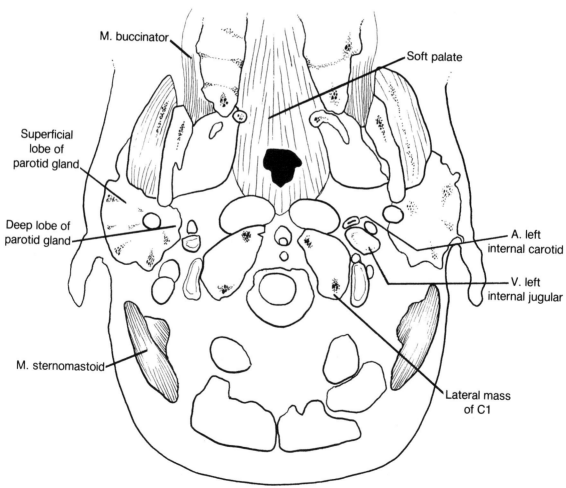

M. buccinator

Soft palate

Superficial
lobe of
parotid gland

Deep lobe of
parotid gland

A. left
internal carotid

V. left
internal jugular

M. sternomastoid

Lateral mass
of C1

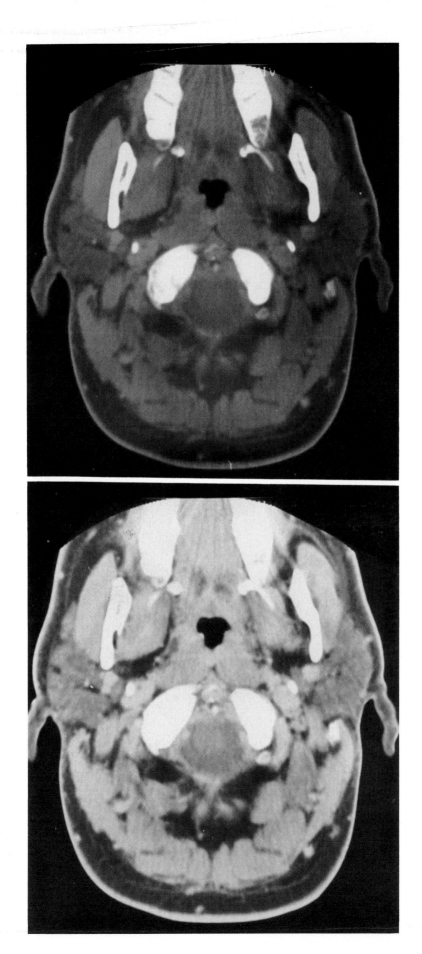

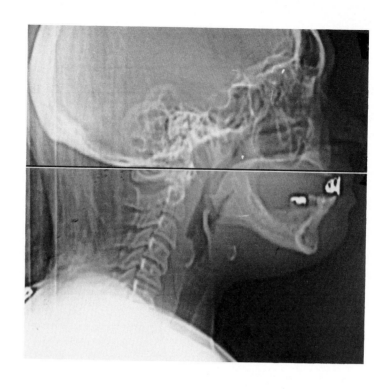

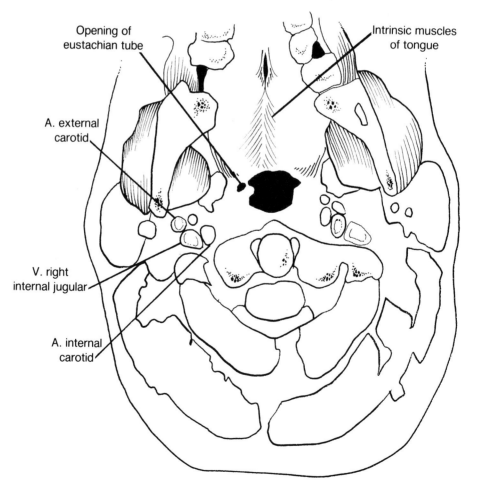

Opening of
eustachian tube

Intrinsic muscles
of tongue

A. external
carotid

V. right
internal jugular

A. internal
carotid

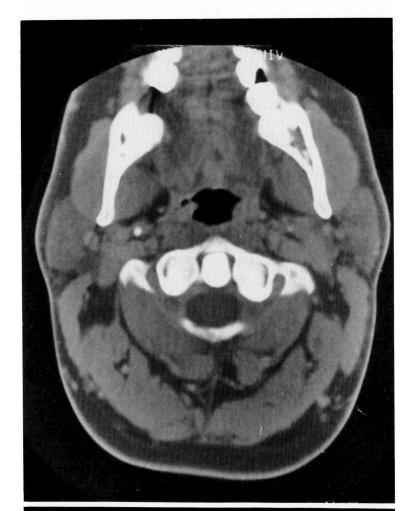

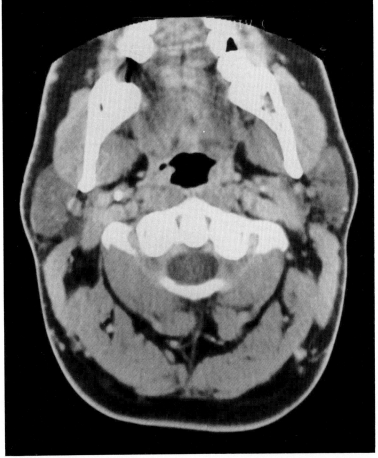

Oropharynx

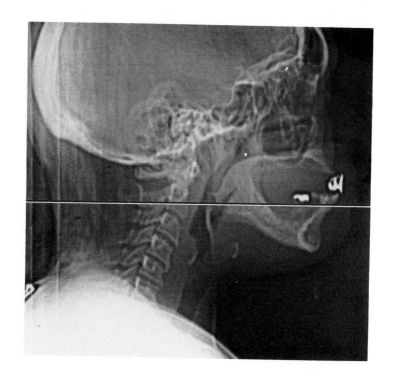

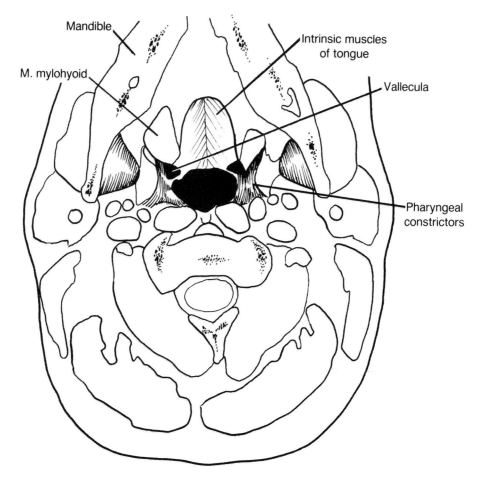

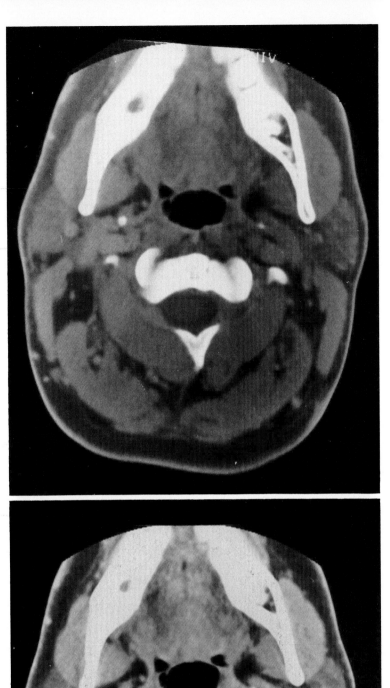

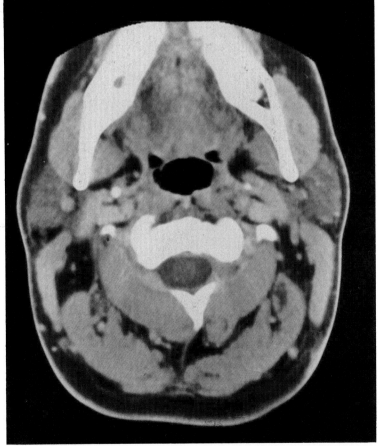

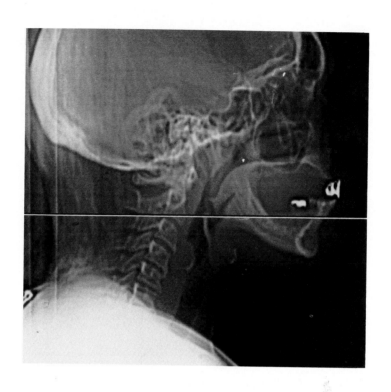

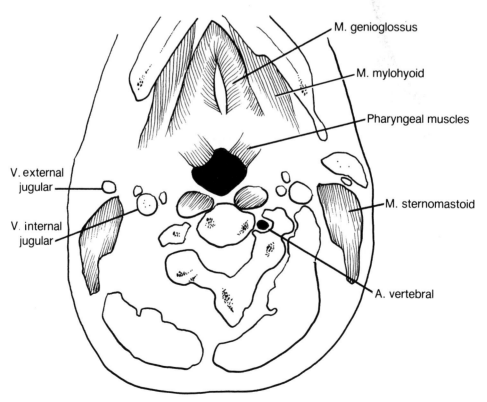

M. genioglossus

M. mylohyoid

Pharyngeal muscles

V. external
jugular

V. internal
jugular

M. sternomastoid

A. vertebral

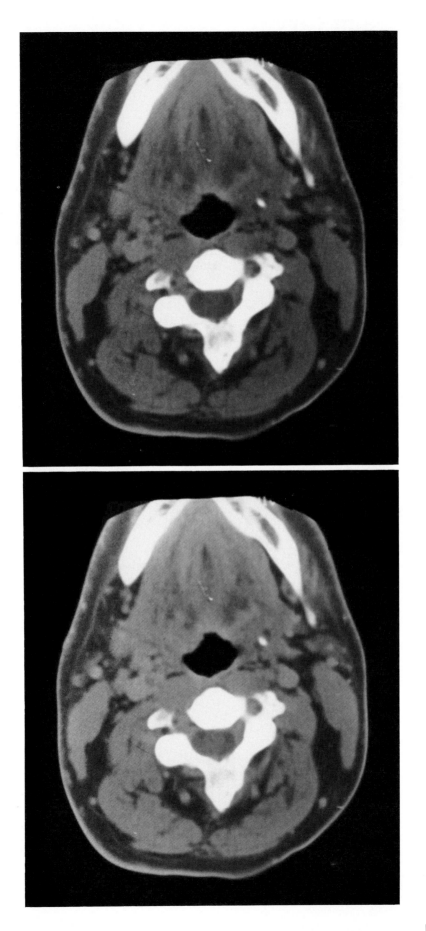

Hypopharynx and Larynx

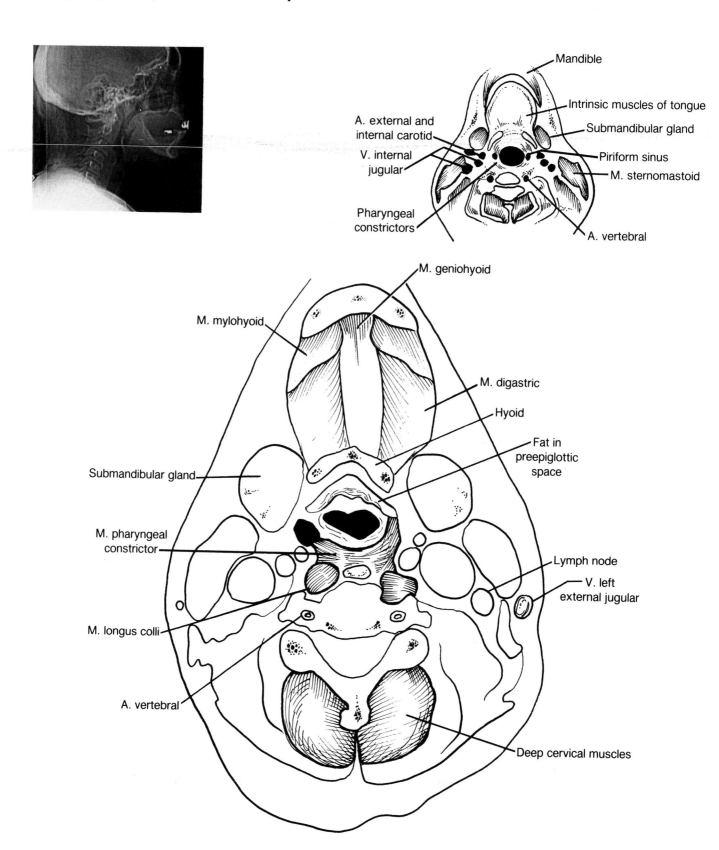

Mandible

Intrinsic muscles of tongue

A. external and internal carotid

Submandibular gland

V. internal jugular

Piriform sinus

M. sternomastoid

Pharyngeal constrictors

A. vertebral

M. geniohyoid

M. mylohyoid

M. digastric

Hyoid

Submandibular gland

Fat in preepiglottic space

M. pharyngeal constrictor

Lymph node

V. left external jugular

M. longus colli

A. vertebral

Deep cervical muscles

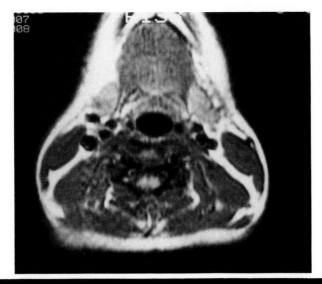

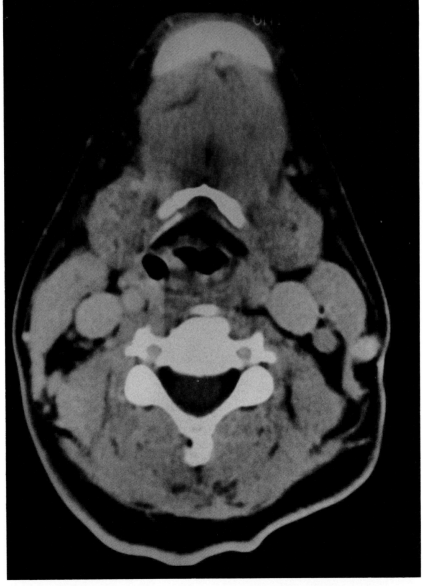

Axial MR (*top*) and CT (*bottom*) at the level of the hyoid.

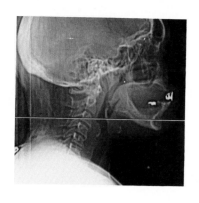

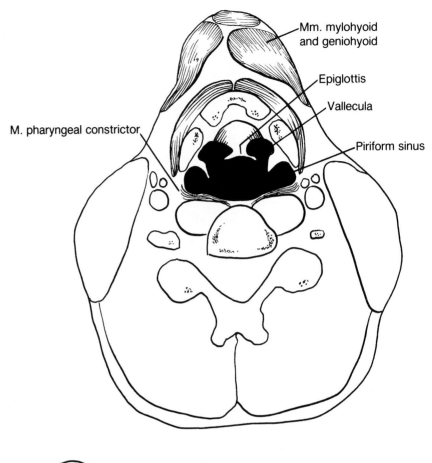

Mm. mylohyoid
and geniohyoid

Epiglottis

Vallecula

Piriform sinus

M. pharyngeal constrictor

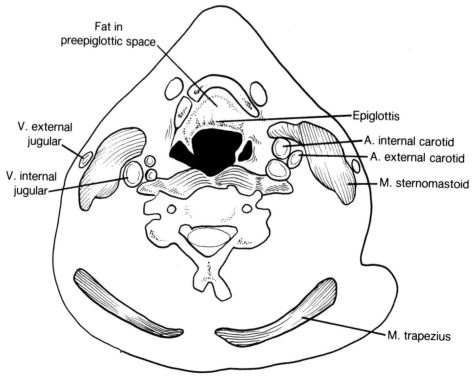

Fat in
preepiglottic space

V. external
jugular

V. internal
jugular

Epiglottis

A. internal carotid

A. external carotid

M. sternomastoid

M. trapezius

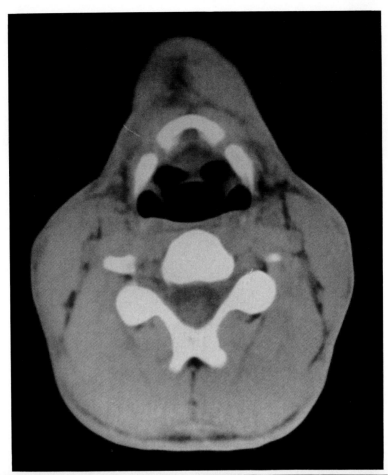

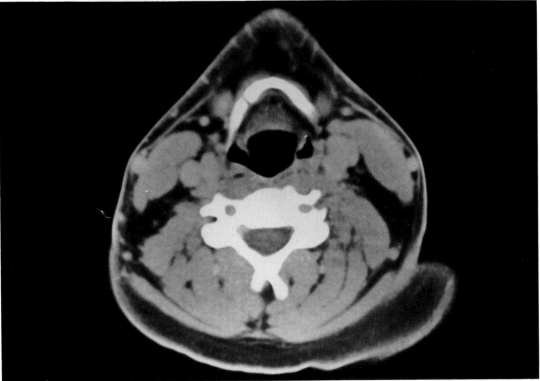

Sections through the hyoid in different individuals; the lower one is at a slightly more caudal level.

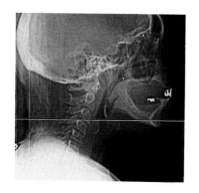

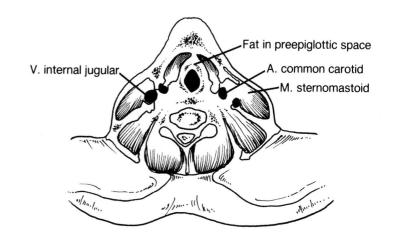

V. internal jugular

Fat in preepiglottic space

A. common carotid

M. sternomastoid

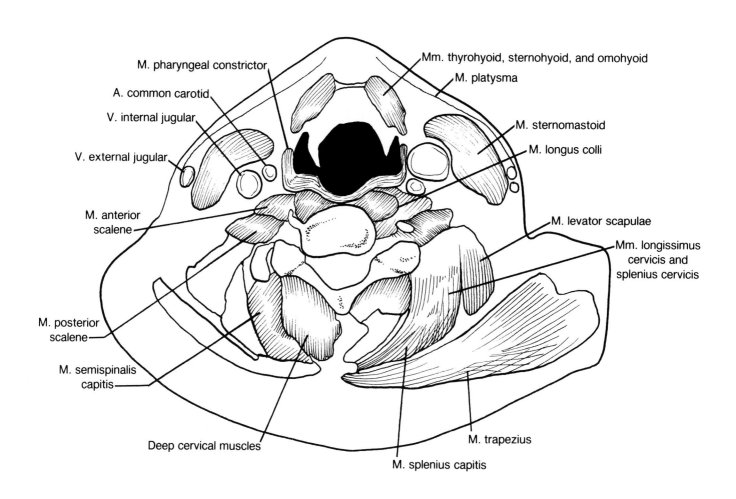

M. pharyngeal constrictor

Mm. thyrohyoid, sternohyoid, and omohyoid

M. platysma

A. common carotid

V. internal jugular

M. sternomastoid

V. external jugular

M. longus colli

M. anterior scalene

M. levator scapulae

Mm. longissimus cervicis and splenius cervicis

M. posterior scalene

M. semispinalis capitis

Deep cervical muscles

M. trapezius

M. splenius capitis

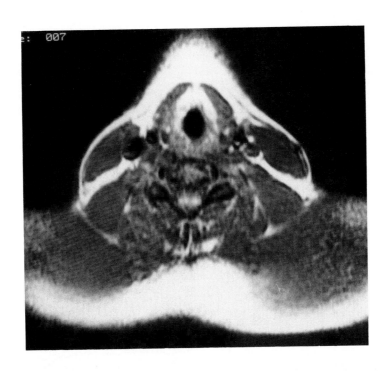

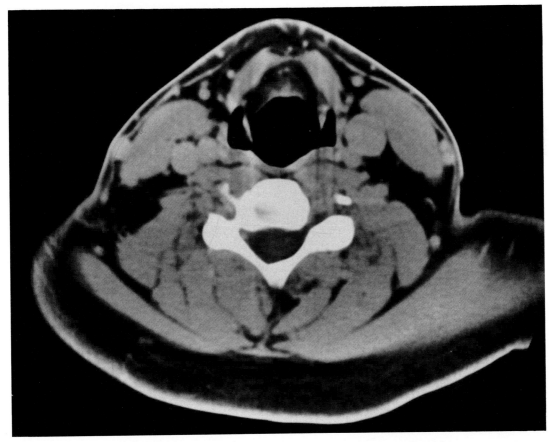

Axial MR (*top*) and CT (*bottom*) just caudal to the hyoid.

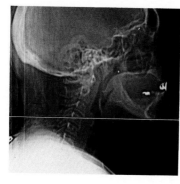

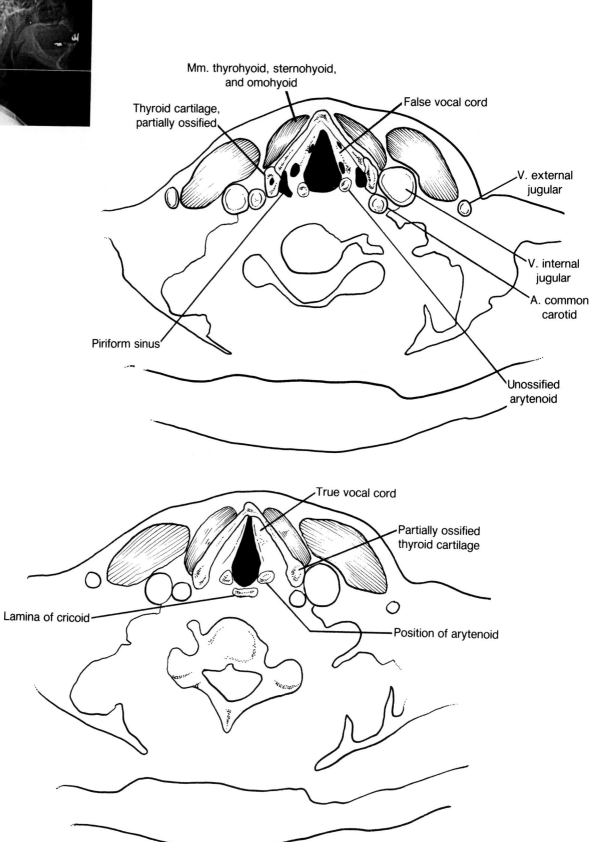

Mm. thyrohyoid, sternohyoid, and omohyoid

Thyroid cartilage, partially ossified

False vocal cord

V. external jugular

V. internal jugular

A. common carotid

Piriform sinus

Unossified arytenoid

True vocal cord

Partially ossified thyroid cartilage

Lamina of cricoid

Position of arytenoid

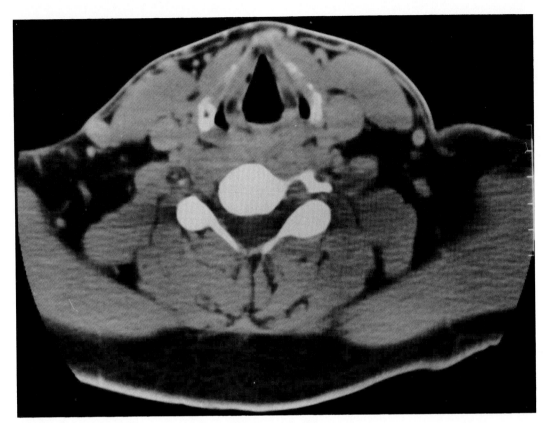

Plane of the false cords.

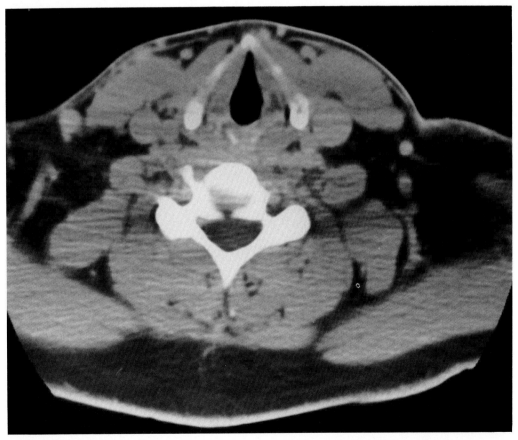

Slightly more caudal level than above, through the plane of the true vocal cords.

Lower Neck

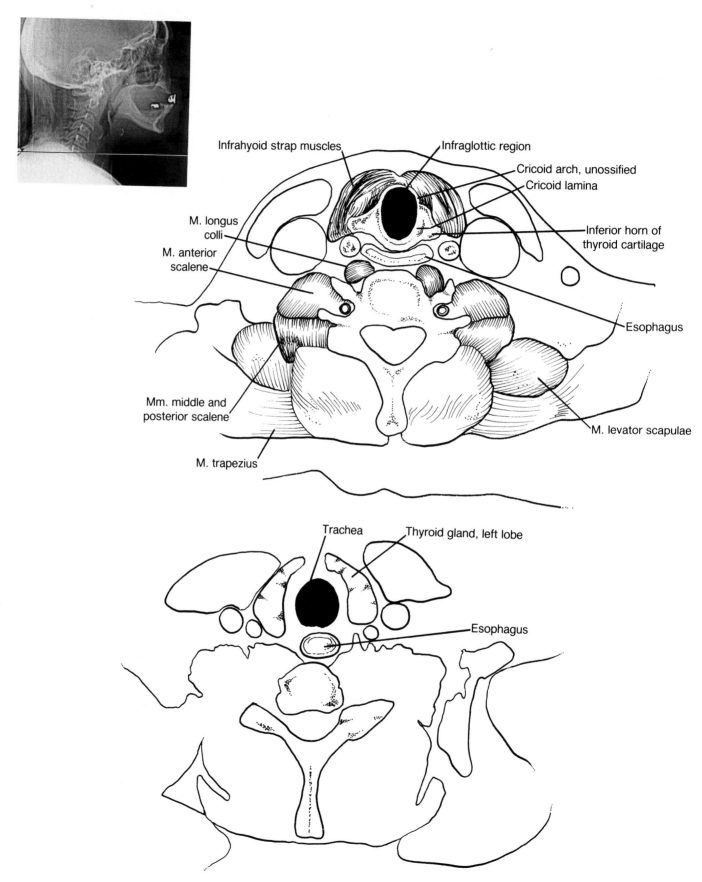

Infrahyoid strap muscles

Infraglottic region

Cricoid arch, unossified

Cricoid lamina

M. longus colli

M. anterior scalene

Inferior horn of thyroid cartilage

Esophagus

Mm. middle and posterior scalene

M. levator scapulae

M. trapezius

Trachea

Thyroid gland, left lobe

Esophagus

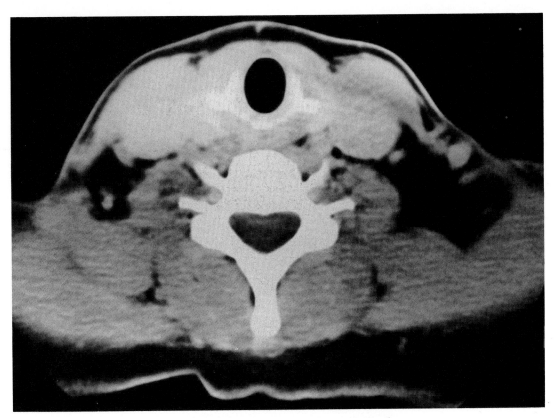

The level of the cricoid cartilage.

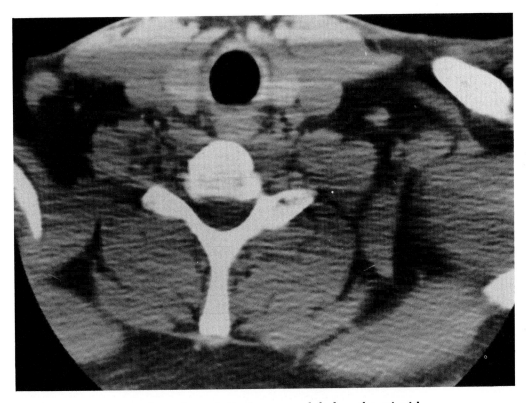

A plane through the lower neck below the cricoid.

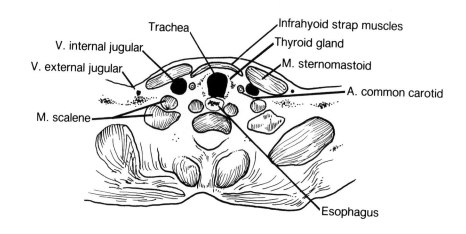

V. internal jugular
V. external jugular
Trachea
Infrahyoid strap muscles
Thyroid gland
M. sternomastoid
A. common carotid
M. scalene
Esophagus

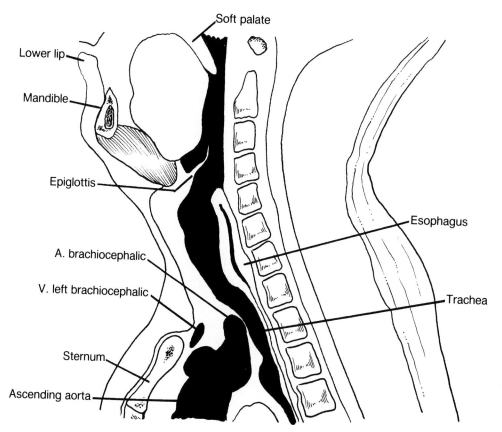

Soft palate
Lower lip
Mandible
Epiglottis
A. brachiocephalic
V. left brachiocephalic
Sternum
Ascending aorta
Esophagus
Trachea

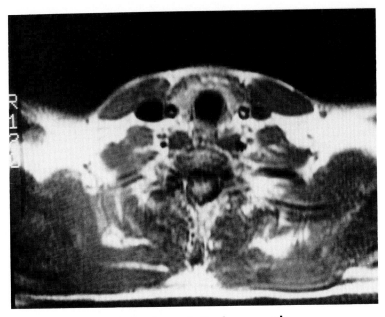

Axial MR through the lower neck.

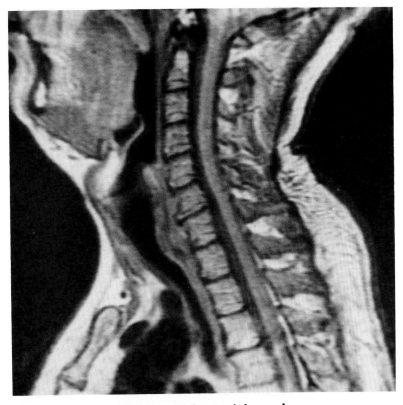

Midline sagittal MR of the neck.

Suggested Readings

Skull and Brain

Alfidi RA, Haaga JR (eds): Magnetic resonance imaging. *Radiol Clin North Am* 22: 763–969, 1984.

Baker HL: The clinical usefulness of routine coronal and sagittal reconstruction in cranial computed tomography. *Radiology* 140:1–9, 1981.

Berman S, Hayman LA, Hinck VC: Correlation of CT cerebral vascular territories with function. III. Middle cerebral artery. *AJNR* 5:161–166, 1984.

Berman SA, Hayman LA, Hinck V: Correlation of CT cerebral vascular territories with function. I. Anterior cerebral artery. *AJNR* 1:259–263, 1980.

Berns TF, Daniels DL, Williams AL, et al: Mesencephalic anatomy: Demonstration by computed tomography. *AJNR* 2:65–67, 1981.

Bradley WG, Adey WR, Hasso AN: *Magnetic Resonance Imaging of the Brain, Head, and Neck: A Text-Atlas.* Rockville, MD, Aspen Systems Corporation, 1985.

Chakeres DW, Kapila A: Brainstem and related structures: Normal CT anatomy using direct longitudinal scanning with Metrizamide cisternography. *Radiology* 149:709–715, 1983.

Daniels DL, Haughton VM, Williams AL, et al: The flocculusin computed tomography. *AJNR* 2:227–229, 1981.

Daniels DL, Haughton VM, Williams AL, et al: Computed tomography of the optic chiasm. *Radiology* 137:123–127, 1980.

Daniels DL, Herfkins R, Gager WE, et al: Magnetic resonance imaging of the optic nerves and chiasm. *Radiology* 152:79–83, 1984.

Daniels DL, Williams AL, Haughton VM: Computed tomography of the medulla. *Radiology* 145:63–69, 1982.

Gonzalez CF, Grossman CB, Masdeu JC (eds): *Head and Spine Imaging.* New York, Wiley, 1985.

Haaga JR, Alfidi RJ (eds): *Computed Tomography of the Brain, Head, and Neck.* St. Louis, C.V. Mosby, 1985.

Hayman LA, Berman SA, Hinck VC: Correlation of CT cerebral vascular territories with function: II. Posterior cerebral artery. *AJNR* 2:219–225, 1981.

Hayward RW, Naeser M, Zatz LM: Cranial computed tomography in aphasia. *Radiology* 123:653–660, 1977.

Huckman MS, Russell EJ: Selecting the optimal plane for CT examination of the base of the skull. *AJNR* 5:333–334, 1984.

Kapila A, Chakeres DW, Blanco E: The Meckel cave: Computed tomographic study. Part 1: Normal anatomy. *Radiology* 152:425–433, 1984.

Koehler PR, Haughton VM, Daniels DL, et al: MR measurements of normal and pathologic brainstem diameters. *AJNR* 6:425–427, 1985.

Latchaw RE (ed): *Computed Tomography of the Head, Neck, and Spine.* Chicago, Year Book Medical Publishers, 1985.

Lee SH, Rao K: *Cranial Computed Tomography.* New York, McGraw-Hill, 1983.

LeMasters DL, Watanabe TJ, Chambers EF, et al: Multiplanar Metrizamide enhanced CT imaging of the foramen magnum. *AJNR* 3:485–494, 1982.

Manelfo C, Clanet M, Gigaud M, et al: Internal capsule: Normal anatomy and ischemic changes demonstrated by computed tomography. *AJNR* 2:149–155, 1981.

Margulis AR, Higgins CB, Kaufman L, et al: *Clinical Magnetic Resonance Imaging.* San Francisco, Radiology Research and Education Foundation, University of California at San Francisco, 1983.

Mawad ME, Silver AJ, Hilal SK, Ganti SR: Computed tomography of the brain stem with intrathecal Metrizamide. Part 1: The normal brain stem. *AJNR* 4:1–11, 1983.

Naidich TP, Leeds NE, Kricheff II, et al: The tentorium in axial section. I. Normal CT appearance and non-neoplastic pathology. *Radiology* 123:631–638, 1977.

New PF, Scott WR: *Computed Tomography of the Brain and Orbit (EMI Scanning).* Baltimore, Williams & Wilkins, 1975.

Newton TH, Potts DG: *Advanced Imaging Techniques*, vol. 2 of Modern Neuroradiology. San Anselmo, CA, Clavadel Press, 1983.

Palacios E, Fine M, Haughton V: *Multiplanar Anatomy of the Head and Neck For Computed Tomography*. New York, Wiley, 1981.

Quisling RG, Lotz PR: *Correlative Neuroradiology. Intracranial Radiographic Analysis with Computed Tomography, Angiography and Magnetic Resonance Imaging*, ed 2. New York, Wiley, 1985.

Shapiro R: *Radiology of the Normal Skull*. Chicago, Year Book Medical Publishers, 1981.

Sherman JL, Citrin CM: Magnetic resonance demonstration of normal CSF flow. *AJNR* 7:3–6, 1986.

Smoker WR, Price MJ, Keyes WD, et al: High resolution computed tomography of the basilar artery. 1. Normal size and position. *AJNR* 7:55–60, 1986.

Taveras JM, Morello F: *Normal Neuroradiology and Atlas of the Skull, Sinuses, and Facial Bones*. Chicago, Year Book Medical Publishers, 1979.

Weisberg L, Nice C, Katz M: *Cerebral Computed Tomography. A Text-Atlas*, ed 2. Philadelphia, W.B. Saunders, 1984.

Whelan MA, Reede DL, Meisler W, et al: CT of the base of the skull. *Radiol Clin North Am* 22:177–217, 1984.

Williams AL, Haughton V: *Cranial Computed Tomography: A Comprehensive Text*. St. Louis, C.V. Mosby, 1985.

Zimmerman RA, Bilaniuk LT: Age related incidence of pineal calcification by computed tomography. *Radiology* 142:659–662, 1982.

Zimmerman R, Yurberg E, Russell EJ, et al: Falx and interhemispheric fissure on axial CT. 1. Normal anatomy. *AJNR* 3:175–180, 1982.

Sella and Juxtasella

Bonneville JF, Catlin F, Portha C, et al: Computed tomography of the posterior pituitary. *AJNR* 6:889–892, 1985.

Chambers EF, Turski PA, LaMasters D, et al: Regions of low density in the contrast-enhanced pituitary gland: Normal and pathologic processes. *Radiology* 144:109–113, 1982.

Daniels DL, Pech P, Leighton M, et al: Magnetic resonance imaging of the cavernous sinus. *AJNR* 6:187–192, 1985.

Earnest F, McCullough E, Frank DA: Fact or artifact: An analysis of artifact in high resolution computed tomographic scanning of the sella. *Radiology* 140:109–113, 1981.

Hasso AN, Pop PM, Thompson JR, et al: High resolution thin section computed tomography of the cavernous sinus. *Radiographics* 2:83–100, 1982.

Johnson DM, Hopkins RJ, Hanafee WN, et al: The unprotected parasphenoidal carotid artery studied by high resolution computed tomography. *Radiology* 155:137–141, 1985.

Kline L, Acker JD, Donovan-Post MJ, et al: The cavernous sinus: A computed tomographic study. *AJNR* 2:299–305, 1981.

Lee KF, Lin SR: *Neuroradiology of Sellar and Juxtasellar Lesions*. Springfield, IL, Charles C Thomas, 1979.

Mark L, Peck P, Daniels D, et al: The pituitary fossa: A correlative anatomic and MR study. *Radiology* 153:453–457, 1984.

Peyster R, Hoover ED, Adler LP: CT of the normal pituitary stalk. *AJNR* 5:45–47, 1984.

Roppolo HMN, Latchaw RE, Meyer JD, et al: Normal pituitary gland: 1. Macroscopic anatomy–CT correlation. *AJNR* 4:927–936, 1983.

Roppolo HMN, Latchaw RE: Normal pituitary gland: 2. Microscopic anatomy—CT correlation. *AJNR* 4:937–944, 1983.

Seidel FG, Towbin R, Kaufman R: Normal pituitary stalk size in children: CT study. *AJNR* 6:733–738, 1985.

Swartz JD, Russell KB, Basik B, et al: High resolution computed tomography of the intrasellar contents: Normal, near normal and abnormal. *Radiographics* 3:228–247, 1983.

Swartz JD, Russell KB, Basik B, et al: High resolution computed tomographic appearance of the intrasellar contents in women of childbearing age. *Radiology* 147:115–117, 1983.

Taylor S: High resolution computed tomography of the sella. *Radiol Clin North Am* 20:207–236, 1982.

Wiener SN, Rzeszotarski MS, Droege RT, et al: Measurement of pituitary gland height with MR imaging. *AJNR* 6:717–722, 1985.

Wolpert SM, Molitch ME, Goldman JA, et al: Size, shape, and appearance of the normal female pituitary gland. *AJNR* 5:263–267, 1984.

Orbit

Bacon TK, Duchesneau PM, Weinstein MA: Demonstration of the superior ophthalmic vein by high resolution computed tomography. *Radiology* 124:129–131, 1977.

Forbes G: Computed tomography of the orbit. *Radiol Clin North Am* 20:37–49, 1982.

Hammerschlag SB, Hesselink JR, Weber AL: *Computed Tomography of the Eye and Orbit*. Norwalk, CT, Appleton-Century-Crofts, 1983.

Hammerschlag SB, O'Reilly GVA, Naheedy M: Computed tomography of the optic canals. *AJNR* 2:593–594, 1981.

Mafee MF, Pruzansky S, Corrales MM: CT in the evaluation of the orbit and bony interorbital distance. *AJNR* 7:265–269, 1986.

Moseley IF, Sanders MD: *Computerized Tomography in Neuro-ophthalmology*. Philadelphia, W.B. Saunders, 1982.

Peyster RG, Hoover ED: *Computerized Tomography in Orbital Disease and Neuro-ophthalmology*. Chicago, Year Book Medical Publishers, 1984.

Russell EJ, Czervionke L, Huckman M, et al: CT of the inferomedial orbit and the lacrimal drainage apparatus: Normal and pathologic anatomy. *AJNR* 6:759–766, 1985.

Schenck JF, Hart HR, Foster TH, et al: Improved MR Imaging of the orbit at 1.5 T with surface coils. *AJNR* 6:193–196, 1985.

Sobel DF, Mills C, Char D, et al: NMR of the normal and pathologic eye and orbit. *AJNR* 5:345–350, 1984.

Unsold R, DeGroot J, Newton TH: Images of the optic nerve: Anatomic-CT correlation. *AJNR* 1:317–323, 1980.

Weinstein MA, Modic MT, Risius B, et al: Visualization of the arteries, veins and nerves of the orbit by sector computed tomography. *Radiology* 138:83–87, 1981.

Paranasal Sinuses and Nasopharynx

Bergeron RT, Osborne AG, Som PM (eds): *Head and Neck Imaging Excluding the Brain*. St. Louis, C.V. Mosby, 1984.

Braun IF, Hoffman JC: Computed tomography of the buccomasseteric region. 1. Anatomy. *AJNR* 5:605–610, 1984.

Curtin Williams R: Computed tomography of the pterygopalatine fossa. *Radiographics* 5:429–440, 1985.

Daniels DL, Rauschning W, Loras J, et al: Pterygopalatine fossa: Computed tomography studies. *Radiology* 149:511–516, 1983.

Dillon WP, Mills CM, Kjos B, et al: Magnetic resonance imaging of the nasopharynx. *Radiology* 152:731–738, 1984.

Dodd G, Jing BS: *Radiology of the Nose, Paranasal Sinuses, and Nasopharynx*. Baltimore, Williams & Wilkins, 1977.

Gentry LR, Manor WF, Turski PA, et al: High resolution CT analysis of facial struts in trauma. 1. Normal anatomy. *AJNR* 140:523–532, 1983.

Hanafee W, Mancuso A: *Introductory Workbook for CT of the Head and Neck*. Baltimore, Williams & Wilkins, 1984.

Mancuso A, Bohman L, Hanafee W, et al: Computed tomography of the nasopharynx: Normal and variants of the normal. *Radiology* 137:113–121, 1980.

Mancuso A, Hanafee WH: *Computed Tomography and Magnetic Resonance Imaging of the Head and Neck*, ed 2. Baltimore, Williams & Wilkins, 1985.

Shatz CJ, Becker TS: Normal CT anatomy of the paranasal sinuses. *Radiol Clin North Am* 22:107–118, 1984.

Silver AJ, Sane P, Hilal SK: CT of the nasopharyngeal region: Normal and pathologic anatomy. *Radiol Clin North Am* 22:161–176, 1984.

Terrier F, Weber W, Ruenfenacht D. Porcellini B: Anatomy of the ethmoid: CT, endoscopic and macroscopic. *AJNR* 6:77–84, 1985.

Towbin R, Dunbar JS: The paranasal sinuses in children. *Radiographics* 2:253–279, 1982.

Valvasori G, Potter GD, Hanafee WN, et al: *Radiology of the Ear, Nose, and Throat*. Philadelphia, W.B. Saunders, 1982.

Temporal Bone

Bhimani S, Virapongse C, Sarwar M: High resolution computed tomographic appearance of the normal cochlear aqueduct. *AJNR* 5:715–720, 1984.

Chakeres DW: CT of ear structures: A tailored approach. *Radiol Clin North Am* 22:3–14, 1984.

Chakeres DW, Kapila A: Normal and pathologic radiographic anatomy of the motor innervation of the face. *AJNR* 5:591–597, 1984.

Chakeres DW, Spiegel PK: A systematic technique for comprehensive evaluation of the temporal bone by computed tomography. *Radiology* 146:97–106, 1983.

Daniels DL, Schenck JF, Foster T, et al: Magnetic resonance imaging of the jugular foramen. *AJNR* 6:699–703, 1985.

Daniels DL, Schenck JF, Foster T, et al: Surface coil magnetic resonance imaging of the internal auditory canal. *AJNR* 6:487–490, 1985.

Daniels DL, Williams AL, Haughton VM: Jugular foramen: Anatomic and computed tomographic study. *AJNR* 4:1227–1232, 1983.

Koenig H, Lenz M, Sauter R: Temporal bone region: High resolution MR imaging using surface coils. *Radiology* 159:191–194, 1986.

Lo WWM, Solti-Bohman LG: High resolution CT of the jugular foramen: Anatomy and vascular variants and anomalies. *Radiology* 150:743–747, 1984.

New PF, Bachow TB, Wismer GL, et al: MR imaging of the acoustic nerves and small acoustic neuromas at 0.6T: Prospective study. *AJNR* 6:165–170, 1985.

Swartz JD: High resolution computed tomography of the middle ear and mastoid. Part I: Normal radioanatomy including normal variations. *Radiology* 148:449–454, 1983.

Taylor S: The petrous temporal bone (including the cerebellopontine angle). *Radiol Clin North Am* 20:67–86, 1982.

Valvanis A, Kubik S, Oguz M: Exploration of the facial nerve canal by high resolution computed tomography. *Neuroradiology* 24:139–147, 1983.

Virapongse C, Rothman SLG, Kier EL, et al: Computed tomographic anatomy of the temporal bone. *AJNR* 3:379–389, 1982.

Virapongse C, Sarwar M, Bhimani S, et al: Computed tomography of the temporal bone pneumatization: Normal pattern and morphology. *AJNR* 6:551–559, 1985.

Viraspongse C, Sarwar M, Bhimani S, et al: Petrosquamosal suture and septum. *AJNR* 6:561–568, 1985.

Viraponge C, Sarwar M, Sasaki C, et al: High resolution computed tomography of the osseus external auditory canal. 1. Normal anatomy. *J Comput Assist Tomogr* 7:486–492, 1983.

Zonneveld FW, Van Waes PFG, Demsa H, et al: Direct multiplanar computed tomography of the temporal bone. *Radiographics* 3:400–449, 1983.

Spine

Anand AK, Lee BCP: Plain and Metrizamide CT of lumbar disk disease: Comparison with myelography. *AJNR* 3:567–571, 1982.

Badami JP, Norman D, Barbaro N, et al: Metrizamide CT myelography in cervical myelopathy and radiculopathy: Correlation with conventional myelography and surgical findings. *AJNR* 6:59–64, 1985.

Carrera GF, Haughton VM, Syvertsen A, et al: Computed tomography of the lumbar facet joints. *Radiology* 134:145–148, 1980.

Cohen BA, Lanzieri CF, Mendelson D, et al: CT evaluation of the greater sciatic foramen in patients with sciatica. *AJNR* 7:337–342, 1986.

Daniels DL, Williams AL, Haughton VM: Computed tomography of the articulations and ligaments at the occipito-atlantal region. *Radiology* 146:709–716, 1983.

Donovan-Post MJ (ed): *Computed Tomography of the Spine*. Baltimore, Williams & Wilkins, 1984.

Dowart RH, DeGroot J, Sauerland EK, et al: Computed tomography of the lumbosacral spine: Normal anatomy, anatomic variants and pathologic anatomy. *Radiographics* 2:459–499, 1982.

Dublin AB, McGahan JP, Reid MH: The value of computed tomographic Metrizamide myelography in the neuroradiological evaluation of the spine. *Radiology* 146:79–86, 1983.

Genant HK (ed): *Spine Update 1984*. San Francisco, University of California at San Francisco, 1983.

Genant HK, Chafetz N, Helms CA (eds): *Computed Tomography of the Lumbar Spine*. San Francisco, University of California at San Francisco, 1982.

Grogan J, Daniels DL, Williams AL, et al: The normal conus medullaris: CT criteria for recognition. *Radiology* 151:661–664, 1984.

Han JS, Kaufman B, Saba JY, et al: NMR imaging of the spine. *AJNR* 4:1151–1159, 1983.

Haughton VM, Syvertsen A, Williams AL: Soft tissue anatomy within the spinal canal as seen on computed tomography. *Radiology* 134:649–655, 1980.

Haughton VM, Williams AL: *Computed Tomography of the Spine*. St. Louis, C.V. Mosby, 1982.

Hyman R, Edwards JH, Vacirca SJ, et al: 0.6T MR imaging of the cervical spine: Multislice and multiecho techniques. *AJNR* 6:229–236, 1985.

Jong S, Benson JE, Yoon YS: Magnetic resonance imaging of the spinal column and craniovertebral junction. *Radiol Clin North Am* 22:805–827, 1984.

Lanzieri CF, Hilal SK: Computed tomography of the sacral plexus and sciatic nerve in the greater sciatic foramen. *AJNR* 5:315–318, 1984.

Lee BCP, Deck MDF, Kneeland JB, et al: MR imaging of the craniocervical junction. *AJNR* 6:209–213, 1985.

Maravilla KR, Lesh PH, Weinrab JMC, et al: Magnetic resonance imaging of the lumbar spine with CT correlation. *AJNR* 6:237–245, 1985.

Matozzi F, Moreau JJ, Jiddane M, et al: Correlative anatomic and CT study of the lumbar lateral recess. *AJNR* 4:650–652, 1983.

Meijenhorst GCH: Computed tomography of the lumbar epidural veins. *Radiology* 145:687–691, 1982.

Modic M, Pavlicek W, Weinstein MA, et al: Magnetic resonance imaging of intervertebral disk disease. *Radiology* 152:103–111, 1984.

Modic MT, Weinstein MA, Pavlicek W, et al: Magnetic resonance imaging of the cervical spine: Technical and clinical observations. *AJNR* 15:15–22, 1984.

Newton TH, Potts DG: *Computed Tomography of the Spine and Spinal Cord*, vol 1 of Modern Neuroradiology. San Anselmo, CA, Clavadel Press, 1983.

Norman D, Mills CM, Brant-Zawadzki, M, et al: Magnetic resonance imaging of the spinal cord and canal: Potentials and limitations. *AJNR* 5:9–14, 1984.

Pech P, Daniels DL, Williams AL, et al: The cervical neural foramina: Correlation of microanatomy and CT anatomy. *Radiology* 155:143–146, 1985.

Pech P, Haughton VM: Lumbar intervertebral disk: Correlative MR and anatomic study. *Radiology* 156:699–701, 1985.

Pech P, Haughton VM: CT appearance of unfused ossicles of the lumbar spine. *AJNR* 6:629–631, 1985.

Raskin SP, Keating J: Recognition of lumbar disk disease: Comparison of myelography and computed tomography. *AJNR* 3:215–221, 1982.

Sartoris DJ, Resnick D, Guera J, Jr: Vertebral venous channels: CT appearance and differential considerations. *Radiology* 155:745–749, 1985.

Sobel D, Barkovich A, Mundeloh SH: Metrizamide myelography and postmyelographic computed tomography: Comparative adequacy in the cervical spine. *AJNR* 5:385–390, 1984.

Teplick JG, Haskin ME (eds): CT of the lumbar spine. *Radiol Clin North Am* 21:195–422, 1983.

Whelan MA, Gold RP: Computed Tomography of the sacrum. 1. Normal anatomy. *AJNR* 3:547–554, 1982.

Yeakley JW, Edeiken-Monroe B, Harris JH Jr: *Computerized Tomography of Spinal Trauma and Degenerative Disease*, vol 34 of *Instructional Course Lectures*. American Academy of Orthopedic Surgery, 1985, pp 85–97.

Neck

Bryan NR, Miller RH, Ferreyro RI, et al: CT of the major salivary glands. *AJR* 139:547–554, 1982.

Carter BL, Karmody CS, Blickman JR, et al: CT and sialography: 1. Normal anatomy. *J Comput Assist Tomogr* 5:42–45, 1981.

Carter BL, Ignatow SB: Neck and mediastinal angiography by computed tomography scan. *Radiology* 122:515–516, 1977.

Gamsu G, Mark AS, Webb WR: Computed tomography of the normal larynx during quiet breathing and phonation. *J Comput Assist Tomogr* 5:353–360, 1981.

Halber MD, Daffner RH, Thompson WM: CT of the esophagus. 1. Normal appearance. *AJR* 133:1047–1050, 1979.

Mancuso AA, Harnsberger HR, Muraki AS, et al: Computed tomography of cervical and retropharyngeal lymph nodes: Normal anatomy, variants of normal, and applications in staging head and neck cancer. Part 1: Normal anatomy. *Radiology* 148:709–714, 1983.

Martinez CR, Gayler BW, Kashima H, et al: Computed tomography of the neck. *Radiographics* 3:9–40, 1983.

Muraki AS, Mancuso AA, Harnsberger HR, et al: CT of the oropharynx, tongue base, and floor of the mouth: Normal anatomy and range of variations, and applications in staging carcinoma. *Radiology* 148:725–731, 1983.

Nicholson RL, Kreel L: CT anatomy of the nasopharynx, nasal cavity, paranasal sinuses and infratemporal fossa. *CT* 3:13–23, 1979.

Osborn A, Hanafee WH, Mancuso AA: Normal and pathologic CT anatomy of the mandible. *AJR* 139:555–559, 1982.

Osborn AG, Koehler PR: Computed tomography of the paraspinal musculature: Normal and pathologic anatomy. *AJR* 138:93–98, 1982.

Reede DL, Whelan MA, Bergeron RT: CT of the soft tissue structures of the neck. *Radiol Clin North Am* 22:239–250, 1984.

Reede DL, Whelan MA, Bergeron RT: Computed tomography of the infrahyoid neck. Part 1: Normal anatomy. *Radiology* 145:389–395, 1982.

Silver AJ, Mawad ME, Hilal SK, et al: Computed tomography of the carotid space and related cervical spaces. Part 1: anatomy. *Radiology* 150:723–728, 1984.

Silver AJ, Ganti SR, Hilal SK: Carotid region: Normal and pathologic anatomy on CT. *Radiol Clin North Am* 22:219–238, 1984.

Silverman PM, Korobkin M, Thompson WM, et al: High resolution, thin-section computed tomography of the larynx. *Radiology* 145:723–725, 1982.

Swartz JD, Lansman A, Marlowe FI, et al: High resolution computed tomography. Part 3: The larynx and hypopharynx. *Head Neck Surg* 7:231–242, 1985.

Unger JM, Chintapalli KN: Computed tomography of the parapharyngeal space. *J Comput Assist Tomogr* 7:605–609, 1983.